# The KySS℠ (Keep Your Children/Yourself Safe and Secure) Guide to Child and Adolescent Mental Health Screening, Early Intervention and Health Promotion

**Editor**

Bernadette Mazurek Melnyk, PhD, RN, CPNP/NPP, FAAN, FNAP

**Assistant Editor**

Zendi Moldenhauer, PhD, RN-CS, CPNP/NPP

## A Publication of the National Association of Pediatric Nurse Practitioners (NAPNAP)

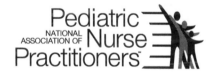

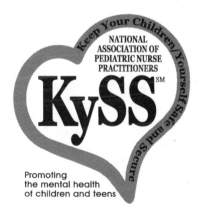

# Dedication

This book is dedicated to all of the children and teens with emotional and/or behavioral problems for whom we have cared, especially those hospitalized in the children and youth inpatient unit at Elmira Psychiatric Center in Elmira, New York, as well as those in our COPE for HOPE, Inc. clinical practice. These children and their families have touched our lives and hearts and have taught us that "rainbows often follow rain." Our lives have been enriched by our experiences with them. We have been blessed to learn from these families and to help them to see a brighter future ahead.

*Bernadette Mazurek Melnyk*                                      *Zendi Moldenhauer*

# TABLE OF CONTENTS

## Section 3
## Anxiety Disorders

## Section 4
## Attention-Deficit/Hyperactivity Disorder (ADHD)

## Section 5
## Eating Disorders

## Section 6
## Grief and Loss

## Section 7
## Mood Disorders

## Section 8
## Marital Separation and Divorce

## Section 9
## Maltreatment

## Section 10
## Sexuality

## Section 11
## Substance Abuse

# The KySS<sup>SM</sup> (Keep your children/yourself Safe and Secure) Guide to Child and Adolescent Mental Health Screening, Early Intervention and Health Promotion

**Editor**

Bernadette Mazurek Melnyk, PhD, RN, CPNP/NPP, FAAN, FNAP
Founder and Director, NAPNAP's KySS Program

**Assistant Editor**

Zendi Moldenhauer, PhD, RN-CS, CPNP/NPP

---

**Contributors**

Linda Alpert-Gillis, PhD
Associate Professor of Psychiatry/Psychology, Pediatrics and Nursing
Director, Child and Adolescent Out-Patient Services Golisano Children's Hospital at Strong
University of Rochester
Rochester, New York
Section: Marital Separation and Divorce

Holly Brown, MS, RN, NPP, CS
Psychiatric Nurse Practitioner
Hillside Children's Center and COPE for HOPE, Inc.
Rochester, New York
Assistant Professor
SUNY Stony Brook School of Nursing
Stony Brook, New York
Doctoral Student and Senior Teaching Associate
University of Rochester School of Nursing
Rochester, New York
Section: Anxiety Disorders

Laura B. Harting, MSW, CSWR
Children's Bereavement Therapist
The Center for Living with Loss Hospice of Central New York
990 Seventh North Street
Liverpool, New York
Section:  Grief and Loss

Elizabeth Hawkins-Walsh, PhD, RN, CPNP
Director, Pediatric Nurse Practitioner Program and Clinical Assistant Professor
The Catholic University of America
Washington, D.C.
Section: Well-Child Visit Handout in Assessing and Screening for Common Mental Health Problems

Neil Herendeen, MD
Associate Professor, General Pediatrics
University of Rochester School of Medicine and Dentistry
Rochester, New York
Section: Reimbursement

Pamela Herendeen, MS, RN-CS, PNP
Senior Nurse Practitioner, Pediatric Nursing
Golisano Children's Hospital at Strong
Rochester, New York
Assistant Professor of Clinical Nursing
University of Rochester School of Nursing
Rochester, New York
Section: Maltreatment

Richard Kriepe, MD
Chair, Department of Adolescent Medicine
Director, Leadership in Education in Adolescent Health
University of Rochester School of Medicine and Dentistry
Rochester, New York
Section: Eating Disorders

Carol Loveland-Cherry, PhD, MPH, RN, FAAN
Professor and Executive Associate Dean for Academic Affairs
University of Michigan School of Nursing
Ann Arbor, Michigan
Section: Substance Abuse

Bernadette Mazurek Melnyk, PhD, RN, CPNP/NPP, FAAN, FNAP
Founder and Director, NAPNAP's KySS Program
Dean and Distinguished Foundation Professor in Nursing
Pediatric and Psychiatric Nurse Practitioner
Arizona State University College of Nursing
Tempe, Arizona
Sections: Assessing and Screening for Common Mental Health Problems, Diagnosing, Managing
and Preventing Mental Health Disorders, Anxiety Disorders, Introduction to Cognitive-Behavior
Skills Building in Brief Interventions, Marital Separation and Divorce

Zendi Moldenhauer, PhD, RN-CS, CPNP/NPP
Pediatric and Psychiatric Nurse Practitioner
Private Practice and COPE for HOPE, Inc.
Rochester, New York
Section: Mood Disorders

Mary Muscari, PhD, CRNP, APRN-BC
Associate Professor of Nursing
University of Scranton
Scranton, Pennsylvania
Section: Violence

Carol Roye, PhD, RN, CPNP
Associate Professor
Hunter College
New York, New York
Section: Sexuality

Naomi A. Schapiro, RN, MS, CPNP
Associate Clinical Professor
Department of Family Health Care Nursing
University of California, San Francisco
Section: Introduction to Motivational Interviewing in Brief Interventions

Daryl Sharp, PhD, RN
Assistant Professor of Nursing
University of Rochester
School of Nursing
Rochester, New York
Section: Tobacco Use among Children and Adolescents in Brief Interventions

Leigh Small, PhD, RN-CS, CPNP
Assistant Professor and Coordinator, Pediatric Nurse Practitioner Program
Arizona State University College of Nursing
Tempe, Arizona
Section:  Eating Disorders

Joy M. Tompkins, MS, RN, PNP
Project Administrator
Pediatric Infectious Disease Division
Department of Pediatrics
SUNY Upstate Medical University
Syracuse, New York
Section:  Grief and Loss

Jane Tuttle, PhD, RN, CPNP
Professor of Clinical Nursing and FNP Program Co-Director
University of Rochester School of Nursing
Rochester, New York
Sections: ADHD and Substance Abuse

Diane Tyler, PhD, RN, CNS, FNP
Associate Professor of Clinical Nursing
University of Texas at Austin
Austin, Texas
Section: Introduction to Motivational Interviewing in Brief Interventions

# Foreword

## The KySS Guide to Child and Adolescent Mental Health Screening, Early Intervention and Health Promotion

I was trained in pediatrics in the early 1950's in a prestigious children's hospital and felt quite competent to deal with the health problems seen in that hospital. At the completion of my training I was offered a position by the head of the department of pediatrics, a very wise and intuitive man, to develop a program to educate pediatricians in the more general aspects of pediatrics. He recognized that the training, based largely on children with diseases serious enough to bring them to this specialized hospital, did not prepare his trainees to be the most effective care givers for the majority of children they would see in their practice. To implement this goal I recruited several hundred low to middle income families living in the area and offered them family focused care, including both preventive as well as curative services, but neither my chief nor I were prepared for the problems these "normal" families brought to us. True they had lots of common medical problems, infections and injuries, and we knew how to care for these. Very soon we recognized that what they really needed and wanted from us was help in raising their children in the rapidly changing cultural environment and help dealing with what we called behavioral problems. Neither they nor we were prepared for this.

We sought help from very experienced psychiatrists and social workers, but while they were helpful, their training and experience was with the more severely disturbed families and hardly any with prevention. Together with the help of other behavioral scientists we evolved a program that focused on caring for the entire family and understanding the cultural, economic and biological factors these families faced. One of the byproducts of our intimate knowledge of these families was the recognition of the inter-relation of psychological stress and common infectious diseases, something labeled in shorthand as "Stress and Strep" [1]. We recognized the problems but we had little to guide us in our care of these families.

A few years later I was given the opportunity to head a department of pediatrics in another city. I was anxious to apply what we had learned from a small group of families to a whole community. Among the initiatives we under took was a random household survey that asked, among other things, what were the main problems these families faced. Ten to fifteen percent identified behavioral problems, a much higher per cent than any physical health problems. We called this phenomenon "the new morbidity. [2]"

These were not new problems; families have always faced problems of behavior with their children but prior to the antibiotic and multiple immunization era these behavioral problems were less pressing or salient for families. In addition, as shown by the national KySS survey, the prevalence today is probably double what we found in the mid 1960's. While we do not know what all the factors are that are behind the rise in problem behaviors among our children, another even greater challenge that emerges from the KySS survey is that only 30 percent of pediatric health care providers screened school age children for mental health problems and this and other studies have demonstrated that a minority of children found to have mental health problems are receiving adequate care. One of the many reasons that primary care clinicians do not screen children for behavioral problems nor initiate therapy when found has been the lack of education of the health professions about these problems. Into that void steps this book to guide the health professional from all disciplines about how to screen for such problems and how to intervene. While the book has been developed by nurses, the authorship includes pediatricians, and is equally relevant for all the professionals who care for children. It emphasizes that for most of these problems an inter- disciplinary group is necessary to provide optimal care.

The book covers a wide range of mental health problems and their precipitating causes. Each follows a similar succinct statement of the problem, provides a number of screening instruments for the clinician to use and discusses the course. While there are some short lists of interventions within several of the sections on specific problems, there is a final section on brief interventions which is very helpful. But to become proficient in interventions most of us will need a good deal of additional training and experience if we are to become proficient interveners.

I hope that this book will find a wide distribution among trainees in the health professions and among seasoned clinicians as well, since most of us have not had this type of information at hand when caring for our patients. In retrospect, what a boon this book would have been 40 years ago to me and my staff as we struggled to help families with their children who had problem behaviors.

Robert J. Haggerty, M.D.
Professor and Chair Emeritus
University of Rochester
School of Medicine and Dentistry

1. Meyer RJ and Haggerty RJ Streptococcal Infections in Families; Factors Altering Susceptibilities. Pediatrics 1962; 29:539-549

2. The Families; Chapter 2. Family Functioning and Family Problems. Pless IB and Satterwhite BB in Child Health and the Community   Haggerty, RJ, Roghmann, KJ, and Pless IB (Eds) 2nd Edition,Transaction Publishers New Brunswick NJ, 1993

# Preface

With 20 to 25% of our nation's children and adolescents affected by mental health/psychosocial morbidities, there has never been a more urgent need for improved mental health screening and promotion as well as early interventions in primary care, school health, and other types of pediatric and adolescent clinical settings. Unfortunately, of the 13 million children and teens in the United States who have mental health problems, approximately 70% do not receive any treatment. Many of the morbidities affecting children and teens in this new millennium are not physical illnesses, but rather a watershed of mental health and psychosocial disorders and risk-taking behaviors. Evidence from studies has indicated that a major factor contributing to the lack of treatment for children with mental health problems has been inadequate screening by primary care providers.

Because of these escalating problems, the National Association of Pediatric Nurse Practitioners (NAPNAP) launched a new national program for children and teens in 2001 called KySS℠ (Keep your children/yourself Safe and Secure), which has a mission of preventing and reducing mental health/psychosocial morbidities in children and youth. Specifically, the KySS Program: (1) educates the public about how to recognize pediatric and adolescent mental health problems, (2) teaches healthcare providers how to screen for and intervene early for these problems, and (3) educates providers and teachers on prevention of these problems by building resiliency, coping skills, and developmental assets in children and teens.

Findings from NAPNAP's national KySS survey conducted with over 1,200 children, teens, and parents from 24 states as part of the KySS program identified that the top 5 worries are: how to cope with the stressful things in their lives; anxiety; depression; self-esteem; and parent-child relationships. Despite the prevalence of these worries, children and parents reported that they seldom discussed their concerns with their primary care providers. In addition, findings from administering the KySS survey to over 650 pediatric healthcare providers across the country indicated that only 30% screened school-aged children for various types of mental health problems on a "nearly always" or "always" basis, and approximately 50% screened teens for these problems at all. When asked about their needs for providing mental health, the providers overwhelmingly cited easy-to-use screening tools and educational support materials for families.

As a result of findings from the KySS national survey and a landmark summit that convened more than 70 pediatric/adolescent and mental health interdisciplinary specialists, NAPNAP has developed a mental health screening and promotion guide to enhance healthcare providers' ability to screen for and intervene early in the treatment of common mental health problems in children and teens. Web-based resources are also included, along with parent and child educational materials to use as part of the KySS guide. The content is organized in a user-friendly format to provide quick and easy access to "nuts and bolts" information about each mental health condition and its corresponding *Diagnostic and Statistical Manual of Mental Disorders* (DSM-IV) criteria, screening tools, and educational handouts for parents as well as school-age children and teens.

We leave you the words of a teen that completed the KySS survey: *"No one ever taught me how to deal with stress until I ended up in a hospital because of my awful temper. I wish someone would have talked to me a long time ago about how anger can be a sign of stress. We need to be taught how to cope in healthy ways before bad stuff happens because it's tough growing up as a kid today."* Another school-age child who completed the survey stated, *"Ask kids if they have ever been abused. Nobody asked me until I tried to kill myself."* Let these words remind us to screen for mental health problems on a daily basis and to talk with children and their families TODAY about how to cope and build resiliency in order to face the multiple stressors of tomorrow.

*Bernadette Mazurek Melnyk*
Bernadette Mazurek Melnyk
Founder and Director,
NAPNAP's KySS Program

*Zendi Moldenhauer*
Zendi Moldenhauer

# Acknowledgments

The vision and beginnings of this guide stemmed from ours and Dr. Leigh Small's work with graduate students in the pediatric primary course that we were team teaching. Therefore, we would like to acknowledge Dr. Small and the following individuals for their outstanding contributions to the vision and first draft of this guide:

Marie Dunn, MS, RN, CPNP
Christine Emmerson, MS, RN, PNP
Kelly Fagan, MS, RN, PNP
Kristina Moss, MS, RN, PNP, NPP
Anita O'Brien, BSN, RN
Nancy Swank, MS, RN, CPNP

In addition, we would like to acknowledge all of the KySS Task Force Chairs over the years (Linda Alpert-Gillis, Michelle Beauchesne, Lisa Bernardo, Holly Brown, Sharon Gullo, Elizabeth Hawkins-Walsh, Pamela Herendeen, Neil Herendeen, Richard Kreipe, Carol Loveland-Cherry, Carol Roye, Leigh Small, Jane Tuttle, Tener Veenema, Judith Vessey), and the KySS Work Group (Michelle Beauchesne, Elizabeth Hawkins-Walsh, Dolores Jones, Mary Muscari), many of whom contributed to this guide, who gave of themselves tirelessly throughout the early years of the program and were instrumental to its successful launch and implementation. We also would like to thank Elizabeth Hawkins-Walsh for her thorough review and critique of the guide. Finally, we would like to recognize and give our appreciation to Dr. Dolores Jones from NAPNAP and Dr. Julie Novak, who have provided outstanding contributions and support to the KySS program, as well as to Lowe's Home Safety Council and the Health Resources Services Administration (HRSA)/Maternal and Child Health Bureau for their funding, which has supported various phases of the program. Because of all of these contributions, the KySS guide has come to fruition.

*Bernadette Mazurek Melnyk*                              *Zendi Moldenhauer*

## Introduction to Assessment and Screening for Common Mental Health Problems

Every encounter with a child or adolescent, whether for a well-child or illness visit, is an opportunity to assess/screen for a mental health or psychosocial problem. Each healthcare encounter also is an excellent time to provide preventive counseling and educational information on how to recognize these conditions early, before the problems become more resistant to early interventions.

Because there is much stigma associated with mental health/behavior problems and parents often feel guilty about them, use of assessment and screening tools can prompt parents to talk about these issues with their healthcare providers. However, it should be remembered that screening tools cannot replace a developmentally sensitive and comprehensive clinical interview. They are especially useful in raising "red flags" signaling that underlying mental health diagnoses may exist. Since fewer than 30% of children with mental health problems are diagnosed and treated, screening is critical for early recognition and intervention.

The following questionnaires in this section of the KySS Guide can be used for the purpose of gaining information on potential mental health/psychosocial problems from families in primary care or other types of pediatric and adolescent clinical settings. Parents can complete the questionnaires while they are waiting for their child's appointment, or the questionnaires can be mailed to them prior to their scheduled visits. It is a good idea to request that parents arrive 15 minutes early if they have not completed the questionnaires so that they have the chance to finish them during their visit.

These questionnaires explore issues that parents may be thinking about or reveal areas of concern. Many of the items on the KySS questionnaires were developed by pediatric and mental health experts who attended the KySS Summit (Melnyk et al., 2003). Once completed, the questionnaires provide healthcare providers with a quick overview of potential or actual mental health/psycho-social issues that need to be more fully assessed during the clinical interview.

# Special Considerations When Interviewing Teens about Mental Health Issues

It is very important to assure teens about confidentiality before the clinical interview begins. Not informing teens of confidentiality is the main reason that they do not confide in their healthcare providers. However, it is also critical to inform them that you cannot hold their information confidential if they tell you that they want to hurt themselves or that someone else has hurt them.

If time for the interview is limited, the HEADSS (Home, Education, Activities, Drugs, Sexuality, Suicide/Depression) Assessment, developed by J.M. Goldenring & E. Cohen, can be very helpful in identifying potential mental health problems

**H**ome (e.g., where is the teen living; who lives in the home; how is the teen getting along with people in the home; has the teen ever run away or been incarcerated?);

**E**ducation (e.g., how is the teen functioning in school in terms of grades, teacher and peer relations, suspensions, missed school days, etc?);

**A**ctivities (e.g., what extracurricular and sports activities is the teen involved in; what does he or she do with his or her friends; etc);

**D**rugs (e.g., which drugs, including IV drugs, alcohol, cigarettes, and caffeine, have been and are used by the teen, his/her family, and friends?);

**S**exuality (e.g., when was the first time the teen had sex; what is the teen's sexual preference; does the teen use contraceptives - and, specifically, does the teen use condoms; how many partners has he or she had; what is the teen's past history of sexually transmitted diseases, pregnancy and abortion, sexual or physical abuse?);

**S**uicide (e.g., has the teen had any suicidal ideations or past history of suicidal attempts; if there have been suicidal ideations, does the teen have a plan?).

# KySS Assessment Questions for
# Parents of Older Infants and Toddlers

Child's Name_____ DOB_____ Age_____

Parent's/Guardian's Name_____ Relationship to Child _____

Because your child's physical as well as mental/emotional health are very important, please complete each of the following questions. We will have the opportunity to talk about some of these issues during your visit. Please indicate which items are most important to talk about today by placing a check mark in front of those items.

1.  What worries or concerns you most about your child's emotions and/or behaviors at this time? _____
    _____

2.  Have there been changes in your family in the past year, such as marital separation, remarriage, move, family illness or death)?  If yes, what?     No   Yes
    _____

3.  Are you afraid of anyone in your home?  If yes, who? _____     No   Yes

4.  Do you ever feel so frustrated that you may hit or hurt your child?     No   Yes

5.  On a scale of 0 (Not at all) to 10 (a lot), how stressed is your child on a day-to-day basis?     _____

6.  Have you been worried about your child being angry, irritable, sad, fearful, or having a change in behavior in the last month? If yes, what is worrying you?     No   Yes
    _____

7.  Do you have any worries about your child being sad?     No   Yes

8.  Are you concerned about your child's weight?  If yes, what concerns you:     No   Yes
    _____

9.  Who usually watches your child when you are not with him or her?_____

10. What is the easiest part about being your child's parent? _____

11. What is the hardest part about being your child's parent? _____

12. What worries you most about your child? _____

13. On a scale of 0 (Not at all) to 10 (a lot), how stressed are you on a day-to-day basis?     _____

14. On a scale of 0 (Not at all) to 10 (a lot), how depressed are you from day-to-day?     _____

15. How do you discipline your child? _____
   _____

16. Do you think that the way that you discipline your child is effective?   No   Yes

17. Do you think that your child has ever been abused? If Yes, when? _____   No   Yes
   _____

18. Has your child ever been through a traumatic or very frightening experience
   (for example, a motor vehicle accident, hospitalization, death of a loved one,
   watching arguments)? If Yes, when and what was the trauma? _____   No   Yes
   _____

19. Has your child ever been diagnosed with an emotional, behavioral, or mental
   health problem?  If yes, what and when? _____   No   Yes

20. Has your child ever been on medication for an emotional, behavioral, or mental
   health problem?  If yes, what medication and when? _____   No   Yes

21. Do you have guns in your home?   No   Yes

22. Are there stressful things that your family has been dealing with recently?
   If yes, what? _____   No   Yes

23. On a scale of 0 (Not at all) to 10 (very), how emotionally connected do you feel
   with your child?   _____

24. On a scale of 0 (very easy) to 10 (very difficult), how is your child's temperament?   _____

25. Does your child have difficulty sleeping?  If yes, what specifically
   (for example, difficulty falling asleep; waking up with nightmares)? _____   No   Yes

26. Does anyone in your home smoke? If yes, who? _____   No   Yes

27. Does anyone in your home use alcohol or drugs to the point that you wish
   they would stop?   No   Yes

28. On a scale of 0 (None) to 10 (a lot), how much arguing goes on in your home?   _____

29. On a scale of 0 (Not at all) to 10 (a lot), do you overprotect your child?   _____

30. On a scale of 0 (Not at all) to 10 (very much so), how satisfied are you
   with being a parent to your child?   _____

31. On a scale of 0 (Not at all) to 10 (very much so), how consistent are you
   in setting limits with your child?   _____

32. Have you or any other of your child's blood relatives ever been diagnosed with
   a mental health disorder?  If yes, who and what? _____   No   Yes

33. What 2 words would you use to best describe your child? _____ _____

# KySS Assessment Questions for Parents of Preschool Children

Child's Name_____ DOB_____ Age_____

Parent's/Guardian's Name_____ Relationship to Child _____

Because your child's physical as well as mental/emotional health are very important, please complete each of the following questions. We will have the opportunity to talk about some of these issues during your visit. Please indicate which items are most important to talk about today by placing a check mark in front of those items.

1.  What worries or concerns you most about your child's emotions and/or behaviors at this time? _____

2.  Have there been changes in your family in the past year, such as marital separation, remarriage, move, family illness or death)?  If yes, what?_____  No  Yes

3.  Are you afraid of anyone in your home?  If yes, who? _____  No  Yes

4.  Do you ever feel so frustrated that you may hit or hurt your child?  No  Yes

5.  On a scale of 0 (Not at all) to 10 (a lot), how much does your child worry on a day-to-day basis? _____

6.  What does your child worry most about? _____

7.  On a scale of 0 (Not at all) to 10 (a lot), how stressed is your child on a day-to-day basis?_____

8.  Have you been worried about your child being angry, irritable, sad, fearful, or having a change in behavior in the last month? If yes, what is worrying you?  No  Yes
    _____

9.  How often does your child complain of headaches or stomachaches?
    a. Never,     b. 1x/month,     c. 2x/month,     d. 1x/week,     c. more that 1x/week

10. Do you have any worries about your child being sad or depressed?  No  Yes

11. Are you concerned about your child's weight? If yes, what concerns you?  No  Yes
    _____

12. Who usually watches your child when you are not with him or her? _____

13. Do you talk about safety with your child?  No  Yes

14. What is the easiest part about being your child's parent?_____

15. What is the hardest part about being your child's parent? _____

16. What worries you most about your relationship with your child? _____

17. On a scale of 0 (Not at all) to 10 (a lot), how stressed are you on a day-to-day basis?  _____

18. On a scale of 0 (Not at all) to 10 (a lot), how depressed are you on a day-to-day basis? _____

19. On a scale of 0 (Not good at all) to 10 (excellent), how does your child cope with stress? _____

20. How do you discipline your child? _____

21. Do you think that the way that you discipline your child is effective?                      No   Yes

22. Do you think that your child has ever been abused? If Yes, when?                      No   Yes
_____

23. Has your child ever been through a traumatic or very frightening experience
(for example, a motor vehicle accident, hospitalization, death of a loved one,
watching arguments)? If Yes, when and what was the trauma? _____      No   Yes
_____

24. Has your child ever been diagnosed with an emotional, behavioral, or mental
health problem? If yes, what and when? _____      No   Yes

25. Has your child ever been on medication for an emotional, behavioral, or mental
health problem? If yes, what medication and when? _____      No   Yes

26. Do you have guns in your home?                      No   Yes

27. Are there stressful things that your family has been dealing with recently?
If yes, what? _____      No   Yes

28. On a scale of 0 (poor) to 10 (excellent), how is your child's self-esteem? _____

29. On a scale of 0 (Not at all) to 10 (very), how emotionally connected do
you feel with your child? _____

30. On a scale of 0 (very difficult) to 10 (very easy), how is your child's temperament? _____

31. Does your child have difficulty sleeping? If yes, what specifically (for example,
difficulty falling asleep; waking up with nightmares)? _____      No   Yes

32. Does anyone in your home smoke? If yes, who? _____      No   Yes

33. Does anyone in your home use alcohol or drugs to the point that you wish
they would stop?                      No   Yes

34. On a scale of 0 (None) to 10 (a lot), how much arguing goes on in your home? _____

35. On a scale of 0 (Not good) to 10 (very good), how well does your child get
along with his/her peers or friends? _____

36. On a scale of 0 (Not at all) to 10 (a lot), do you overprotect your child? _____

37. On a scale of 0 (Not at all) to 10 (very much so), how satisfied are you with
being a parent to your child? _____

38. On a scale of 0 (Not at all) to 10 (very much so), are you consistent in setting
limits with your child? _____

39. Is your child ever cruel to animals?                      No   Yes

# KySS Assessment Questions
## For Parents of School-Age Children and Teens

Child's / Teen's Name_____ DOB_____ Age_____

Parent's/Guardian's Name_____ Relationship to Child _____

Because your child's physical as well as mental/emotional health are very important, please complete each of the following questions. We will have the opportunity to talk about some of these issues during your visit. Please indicate which items are most important to talk about today by placing a check mark before those items.

1.  What worries or concerns you most about your child's emotions and/or behaviors at this time?_____

2.  Have there been changes in your family in the past year, such as marital separation, remarriage, move, family illness or death)? If yes, what? _____  No  Yes

3.  Are you afraid of anyone in your home? If yes, who? _____  No  Yes

4.  Do you ever feel so frustrated that you may hit or hurt your child?  No  Yes

5.  On a scale of 0 (Not at all) to 10 (a lot), how much does your child worry on a day-to-day basis? _____

6.  What does your child worry most about? _____

7.  On a scale of 0 (Not at all) to 10 (a lot), how stressed is your child on a day-to-day basis? _____

8.  Have you been worried about your child being angry, irritable, sad fearful, or having a change in behavior in the last month? If yes, what is worrying you?  No  Yes

9.  How often does your child complain of headaches or stomachaches?
    a. Never,      b. 1x/month,      c. 2x/month,      d. 1x/week,      c. more that 1x/week

10. Do you have any worries about your child being depressed?  No  Yes

11. If yes, do you ever think that your child thinks about hurting him- or herself?  No  Yes

12. Are you concerned about your child's weight? If yes, what concerns you?  No  Yes

13. Does your child make negative comments about his or her body or weight?  No  Yes

14. Where does your child spend his/her free time? _____

15. Who usually watches your child when you are not with him or her? _____

16. Do you talk about safety with your child?                                    No   Yes

17. What is the easiest part about being your child's parent? _____

18. What is the hardest part about being your child's parent? _____

19. What worries you most about your relationship with your child? _____

20. On a scale of 0 (Not at all) to 10 (a lot), how stressed are you on a day-to-day basis?    _____

21. On a scale of 0 (Not at all) to 10 (a lot), how depressed are you on a
    day-to-day basis?                                                                 _____

22. On a scale of 0 (Not good at all) to 10 (excellent), how does your child
    cope with stress?                                                                 _____

23. How do you discipline your child? _____

24. Do you think that the way that you discipline your child is effective?             No   Yes

25. Has your child ever been through a traumatic or very frightening experience (for
    example, a motor vehicle accident, hospitalization, death of a loved one, rape)?
    If Yes, when and what was the trauma? _____   No   Yes
    _____

26. On a scale of 0 (Not at all) to 10 (a lot), how comfortable do you feel in talking
    with your child about sexuality?                                                   _____

27. Are you worried about your child becoming sexually active?                         No   Yes

28. Are you worried about your child and drug or alcohol use?                          No   Yes

29. Are you worried about your child and cigarette smoking?                            No   Yes

30. Does your child ever get bullied?                                                  No   Yes

31. Has your child ever been diagnosed with an emotional, behavioral, or mental
    health problem?  If yes, what and when? _____   No   Yes

32. Has your child ever been on medication for an emotional, behavioral, or mental
    health problem?  If yes, what medication and when? _____   No   Yes

33. Do you have guns in your home?                                                    No   Yes

34. Are there stressful things that your family has been dealing with recently? If yes, what? _____    No   Yes

35. On a scale of 0 (poor) to 10 (excellent), how is your child's self-esteem?    _____

36. On a scale of 0 (Not at all) to 10 (very), how emotionally connected do you feel with your child?    _____

37. On a scale of 0 (very difficult) to 10 (very easy), how is your child's temperament?    _____

38. Has your child had a recent decline in his or her school performance/grades? If yes, when and what? _____    No   Yes

39. Does your child have difficulty sleeping?  If yes, what specifically (for example, difficulty falling asleep; waking up with nightmares)? _____    No   Yes

40. Does anyone in your home smoke? If yes, who? _____    No   Yes

41. Does anyone in your home use alcohol or drugs to the point that you wish they would stop?    No   Yes

42. On a scale of 0 (None) to 10 (a lot), how much arguing goes on in your home?    _____

43. On a scale of 0 (Not good) to 10 (very good), how well does your child get along with his/her peers or friends?    _____

44. On a scale of 0 (Not at all) to 10 (a lot), do you overprotect your child?    _____

45. On a scale of 0 (Not at all) to 10 (very much so), how satisfied are you with being a parent to your child?    _____

46. On a scale of 0 (Not at all) to 10 (very much so), are you consistent in setting limits with your child?    _____

47. Is your child ever cruel to animals?    No   Yes

48. Have you or any other of your child's blood relatives ever been diagnosed with a mental health disorder?  If yes, who and what?    No   Yes

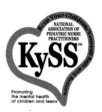

# KySS Assessment Questions for a Specific Emotional or Behavioral Problem

When parents report that they have a specific concern or worry about their child's mental/emotional health or behaviors or that there has been a change in the way the child is functioning at home or school, proceed with the following questions regarding history or background to shed more light on the parent's concern:

1.  **What?**
    a.  What specifically occurs?
    b.  What precipitated it?
    c.  What are the associated symptoms (e.g., headaches, stomachaches)?

2.  **Where?**
    a.  At home and/or school/day care?

3.  **When?**
    a.  Time of day? During a transition?

4.  **Who?**
    a.  Who is with the child when it occurs and who is involved?

5.  **How?**
    a.  How do the parent and others involved react?
    b.  How long has it been going on?

6.  **Why?**
    a.  What makes the parent and child think that this is occurring?


Refer to a mental health specialist if the problem has been persistent, increasing in severity, and/or interfering with functioning at home or in school.

# The Pediatric Symptom Checklist (PSC)
## (M.S. Jellinek & J.M. Murphy)

## Description of the PSC

The PSC is a 1-page questionnaire that lists a range of children's emotional and behavioral concerns as perceived by parents. There is also a youth self-reported version of the scale. The PSC can be easily administered in a pediatric office's waiting room and scored by a receptionist or healthcare provider. A high score indicates likelihood of significant psychosocial dysfunction.

## Age Range: 4 - 18 years

## Psychometric Properties of the PSC

**Instructions for Scoring:** The PSC consists of 35 items that are rated as "never," "sometimes," or "often" present and scored as 0, 1, and 2, respectively. Item scores are summed and the total score is recoded into a dichotomous variable indicating psychosocial impairment. For children aged 6 through 16 years, the cut-off score is 28 or higher. For 4- and 5-year-old children, the PSC cut-off is 24 or higher (Little et al, 1994; Pagano et al, 1996). Items that are left blank by parents are simply ignored (score = 0). If 4 or more items are left blank, the questionnaire is considered invalid.

**How to Interpret the PSC:** A positive score on the PSC suggests the need for further evaluation by a qualified health professional (MD, NP, RN) or mental health professional (PhD, LICSW, Nurse Practitioner of Psychiatry). Both false positives and false negatives occur, and only an experienced clinician should interpret a positive PSC score as anything other than a suggestion that further evaluation may be helpful. Data from past studies using the PSC indicate that 2 out of 3 children who screen positive on the PSC will be correctly identified as having moderate to serious impairment in psychosocial functioning. The one child "incorrectly" identified usually has at least mild impairment, although a small percentage of children turn out to have very little actually wrong with them (e.g., an adequately functioning child of an overly anxious parent). Data on PSC-negative screens indicate 95% accuracy, which still suggest that 1 out of 20 children rated as functioning adequately may actually be impaired. The inevitability of both false-positive and false-negative screens underscores the importance of experienced clinical judgment in interpreting PSC scores. Therefore, it is especially important for parents or other lay persons who administer the form to consult with a licensed professional if their child receives a PSC-positive score.

**Validity:** Using a receiver operating characteristic curve, Jellinek, Murphy, Robinson, and colleagues (1988) found that a PSC cut-off score of 28 has a specificity of 0.68 and a sensitivity of 0.95 when compared with clinicians' ratings of children's psychosocial dysfunction.

**Reliability:** Test retest reliability of the PSC ranges from $r = 0.84$-$0.91$. Over time, case/not case classification ranges from 83%-87%. (Jellinek & Murphy, 1988; Murphy et al, 1992).

**Inter-item Analysis:** Studies (Murphy & Jellinek, 1985; Murphy, Ichinose, Hicks, et al, 1996) also indicate strong internal consistency reliability (Cronbach's alpha = 0.91) of the PSC items and highly significant ($p < 0.0001$) correlations between individual PSC items and positive PSC screening scores.

**Qualifications for Use of the PSC:** The training required may differ according to the ways in which the data are to be used. Professional school (e.g., medicine or nursing) or graduate training in psychology of at least the Master's degree level would ordinarily be expected. However, no amount of prior training can substitute for professional maturity, a thorough knowledge of clinical research methodology, and supervised training in working with parents and children. There are no special qualifications for scoring.

**Source:** Jellinek, M.S., Murphy, J.M., Robinson, J., et al. (1988). Pediatric Symptom Checklist: Screening school age children for psychosocial dysfunction. *Journal of Pediatrics*, 112:201-209. The PSC is one of only a few public domain measures and can be downloaded in English or Spanish at: http://psc.partners.org/, free of charge.

*From: Pediatric Development and Behavior Online, available at http://www.dbpeds.org*

The PSC is in the public domain and can be downloaded for use at http://psc.partners.org.

**Please note:** It is suggested that the Child Behavior Checklist (CBCL) be administered if a positive score is found on the PSC (see information on the CBCL that follows the PSC in this guide).

# Pediatric Symptom Checklist

Child's Name_____          Record Number_____

Today's Date_____          Filled out by_____

Date of Birth_____

**Please mark under the heading that best fits your child:**

|  | Never | Sometimes | Often |
|---|:---:|:---:|:---:|
| 1. Complains of aches/pains | ❑ | ❑ | ❑ |
| 2. Spends more time alone | ❑ | ❑ | ❑ |
| 3. Tires easily, has little energy | ❑ | ❑ | ❑ |
| 4. Fidgety, unable to sit still | ❑ | ❑ | ❑ |
| 5. Has trouble with a teacher | ❑ | ❑ | ❑ |
| 6. Less interested in school | ❑ | ❑ | ❑ |
| 7. Acts as if driven by a motor | ❑ | ❑ | ❑ |
| 8. Daydreams too much | ❑ | ❑ | ❑ |
| 9. Distracted easily | ❑ | ❑ | ❑ |
| 10. Is afraid of new situations | ❑ | ❑ | ❑ |
| 11. Feels sad, unhappy | ❑ | ❑ | ❑ |
| 12. Is irritable, angry | ❑ | ❑ | ❑ |
| 13. Feels hopeless. | ❑ | ❑ | ❑ |
| 14. Has trouble concentrating | ❑ | ❑ | ❑ |
| 15. Has less interest in friends | ❑ | ❑ | ❑ |
| 16. Fights with others. | ❑ | ❑ | ❑ |
| 17. Absent from school | ❑ | ❑ | ❑ |
| 18. School grades dropping | ❑ | ❑ | ❑ |
| 19. Is down on him or herself | ❑ | ❑ | ❑ |
| 20. Visits doctor with doctor finding nothing wrong | ❑ | ❑ | ❑ |
| 21. Has trouble sleeping | ❑ | ❑ | ❑ |
| 22. Worries a lot | ❑ | ❑ | ❑ |
| 23. Wants to be with you more than before | ❑ | ❑ | ❑ |
| 24. Feels he or she is bad | ❑ | ❑ | ❑ |
| 25. Takes unnecessary risks | ❑ | ❑ | ❑ |
| 26. Gets hurt frequently | ❑ | ❑ | ❑ |
| 27. Seems to be having less fun | ❑ | ❑ | ❑ |
| 28. Acts younger than children his or her age | ❑ | ❑ | ❑ |
| 29. Does not listen to rules | ❑ | ❑ | ❑ |
| 30. Does not show feelings | ❑ | ❑ | ❑ |
| 31. Does not understand other people's feelings | ❑ | ❑ | ❑ |
| 32. Teases others. | ❑ | ❑ | ❑ |
| 33. Blames others for his or her troubles | ❑ | ❑ | ❑ |
| 34. Takes things that do not belong to him or her | ❑ | ❑ | ❑ |
| 35. Refuses to share | ❑ | ❑ | ❑ |

Total_____

**Other comments**

Does your child have any emotional or behavioral problems for which he/she needs help?
( ) N ( ) Y

Are there any services that you would like your child to receive for these problems?
( ) N ( ) Y

If yes, what services? _____

# Estudio Sobre Adaptacion Social Y Emocional de los Ninos

La salud fisica y emocional son importantes para cada niño. Los padres son los primeros que notan un problema de la conducta emocional o de aprendizaje. Ud puede ayudar a su hijo a obtener el mejor cuidado del doctor por medio de contestar estas preguntas. Favor de indicar cual frase describe a su niño/a.

## Indique cual síntoma mejor describe a su niño/a:

| | NUNCA | ALGUNAS | SEGUIDO |
|---|---|---|---|
| 1. Se queja de dolores y malestares | ❑ | ❑ | ❑ |
| 2. Pasa mucho tiempo solo(a) | ❑ | ❑ | ❑ |
| 3. Se cansa fácilmente, tiene poca energiá | ❑ | ❑ | ❑ |
| 4. Nervioso, incapaz de estarse quieto | ❑ | ❑ | ❑ |
| 5. Tiene problemas con un maestro | ❑ | ❑ | ❑ |
| 6. Menos interesado en la escuela | ❑ | ❑ | ❑ |
| 7. Es incansable | ❑ | ❑ | ❑ |
| 8. Esta muy un sonador | ❑ | ❑ | ❑ |
| 9. Se distrae facilmente | ❑ | ❑ | ❑ |
| 10. Temeroso/a a nuevas situaciónes | ❑ | ❑ | ❑ |
| 11. Se siete triste, infelix | ❑ | ❑ | ❑ |
| 12. Es irritable, enojon | ❑ | ❑ | ❑ |
| 13. Se siente sin esperanzas | ❑ | ❑ | ❑ |
| 14. Tiene problemas para concentrarse | ❑ | ❑ | ❑ |
| 15. Menos interesado en amistades | ❑ | ❑ | ❑ |
| 16. Pelea con otros niños | ❑ | ❑ | ❑ |
| 17. Se ausenta de la escuela a menudo | ❑ | ❑ | ❑ |
| 19. Se critica a si mismo/a | ❑ | ❑ | ❑ |
| 20. Visita al doctor sin que le encuentren nada | ❑ | ❑ | ❑ |
| 21. Tiene problemas para dormir | ❑ | ❑ | ❑ |
| 22. Se preocupa mucho | ❑ | ❑ | ❑ |
| 23. Quiere estar con usted mas que antes | ❑ | ❑ | ❑ |
| 24. Cree que el/ella es malo/a | ❑ | ❑ | ❑ |
| 25. Toma riezgos innecesarios | ❑ | ❑ | ❑ |
| 26. Se lastima frecuentemente | ❑ | ❑ | ❑ |
| 27. Parece divertirse menos | ❑ | ❑ | ❑ |
| 28. Actua mas chico que niños de su propia edad | ❑ | ❑ | ❑ |
| 29. No obedece las reglas | ❑ | ❑ | ❑ |
| 30. No demuestra sus sentimientos | ❑ | ❑ | ❑ |
| 31. No comprende los sentimientos de otros | ❑ | ❑ | ❑ |
| 32. Molesta o se burla de otros | ❑ | ❑ | ❑ |
| 33. Culpa a otros por sus problemas | ❑ | ❑ | ❑ |
| 34. Toma cosas que no le pertenecen | ❑ | ❑ | ❑ |
| 35. Se rehusa a compartir | ❑ | ❑ | ❑ |

**Total**_____

Necesita su nino(a) ayuda con problemas en el comportamiento con problemas emocionales?
___Si ___No

# Pediatric Symptom Checklist - Youth Report (Y-PSC)

Child's Name_____          Record Number_____

Today's Date_____          Filled out by_____

Date of Birth_____
**Please mark under the heading that best fits you:**

|  | Never | Sometimes | Often |
|---|---|---|---|
| 1. Complain of aches or pains | ❏ | ❏ | ❏ |
| 2. Spend more time alone | ❏ | ❏ | ❏ |
| 3. Tire easily, has little energy | ❏ | ❏ | ❏ |
| 4. Fidgety, unable to sit still | ❏ | ❏ | ❏ |
| 5. Have trouble with teacher | ❏ | ❏ | ❏ |
| 6. Less interested in school | ❏ | ❏ | ❏ |
| 7. Act as if driven by motor | ❏ | ❏ | ❏ |
| 8. Daydream too much | ❏ | ❏ | ❏ |
| 9. Distract easily | ❏ | ❏ | ❏ |
| 10. Are afraid of new situations | ❏ | ❏ | ❏ |
| 11. Feel sad, unhappy | ❏ | ❏ | ❏ |
| 12. Are irritable, angry | ❏ | ❏ | ❏ |
| 13. Feel hopeless | ❏ | ❏ | ❏ |
| 14. Have trouble concentrating | ❏ | ❏ | ❏ |
| 15. Less interested in friends | ❏ | ❏ | ❏ |
| 16. Fight with other children | ❏ | ❏ | ❏ |
| 17. Absent from school | ❏ | ❏ | ❏ |
| 18. School grades dropping | ❏ | ❏ | ❏ |
| 19. Down on yourself | ❏ | ❏ | ❏ |
| 20. Visit doctor and finding nothing wrong | ❏ | ❏ | ❏ |
| 21. Have trouble sleeping | ❏ | ❏ | ❏ |
| 22. Worry a lot | ❏ | ❏ | ❏ |
| 23. Want to be with parent more than before | ❏ | ❏ | ❏ |
| 24. Feel that you are bad | ❏ | ❏ | ❏ |
| 25. Take unnecessary risks | ❏ | ❏ | ❏ |
| 26. Get hurt frequently | ❏ | ❏ | ❏ |
| 27. Seem to be having less fun | ❏ | ❏ | ❏ |
| 28. Act younger than children your age | ❏ | ❏ | ❏ |
| 29. Do not listen to rules | ❏ | ❏ | ❏ |
| 30. Do not show feelings | ❏ | ❏ | ❏ |
| 31. Do not understand other people's feelings | ❏ | ❏ | ❏ |
| 32. Tease others | ❏ | ❏ | ❏ |
| 33. Blame others for your troubles | ❏ | ❏ | ❏ |
| 34. Take things that do not belong to you | ❏ | ❏ | ❏ |
| 35. Refuse to share | ❏ | ❏ | ❏ |

**Total_____**

© 1988, M.S. Jellinek and J.M. Murphy, Massachusetts General Hospital.

# CUESTIONARIO (PSC-Y)

La salud fisica y emocional van juntas. Usted pueda ayudar al doctor/a a obtener el mejor servicio posible, contestando unas pocas preguntas acerca de usted. La informacion que nos de es parte de la visita de hov.

## Indique cual síntoma mejor describe a su niño/a:

| | NUNCA | ALGUNAS | SEGUIDO |
|---|---|---|---|
| 1. Se queja de dolores y malestares | ❏ | ❏ | ❏ |
| 2. Pasa mucho tiempo solo(a) | ❏ | ❏ | ❏ |
| 4. Es inquieto(a) | ❏ | ❏ | ❏ |
| 5. Problemas con un maestro(a) | ❏ | ❏ | ❏ |
| 6. Menos interesado en la escuela | ❏ | ❏ | ❏ |
| 7. Es incansable | ❏ | ❏ | ❏ |
| 8. Es muy sonador | ❏ | ❏ | ❏ |
| 9. Se distrae facilmente | ❏ | ❏ | ❏ |
| 10. Temeroso(a) a nuevas situaciónes | ❏ | ❏ | ❏ |
| 11. Se siete triste, infeliz | ❏ | ❏ | ❏ |
| 12. Es irritable, enojon | ❏ | ❏ | ❏ |
| 13. Se siente sin esperanzas | ❏ | ❏ | ❏ |
| 14. Tiene problemas para concentrandose | ❏ | ❏ | ❏ |
| 15. Menos interesado(a) en amigos(as) | ❏ | ❏ | ❏ |
| 16. Pelea con otros niños(as) | ❏ | ❏ | ❏ |
| 17. Falta a la escuela a menudo | ❏ | ❏ | ❏ |
| 18. Estan bejando sus calificaciones | ❏ | ❏ | ❏ |
| 19. Se critica a si mismo(a) | ❏ | ❏ | ❏ |
| 20. Va al doctor y no encuentren nada | ❏ | ❏ | ❏ |
| 21. Tiene problemas para dormir | ❏ | ❏ | ❏ |
| 22. Se preocupa mucho | ❏ | ❏ | ❏ |
| 24. Cree que eres malo(a) | ❏ | ❏ | ❏ |
| 25. Se pone en peligro sin necesidad | ❏ | ❏ | ❏ |
| 26. Se lastima facilmente | ❏ | ❏ | ❏ |
| 27. Parece divertise menos | ❏ | ❏ | ❏ |
| 28. Actua como un nino a su edad | ❏ | ❏ | ❏ |
| 29. No obedece reglas | ❏ | ❏ | ❏ |
| 30. No demuestra sus sentimientos | ❏ | ❏ | ❏ |
| 31. No comprende el sentir de otros | ❏ | ❏ | ❏ |
| 32. Molesta a otros | ❏ | ❏ | ❏ |
| 33. Culpa a otros de sus problemas | ❏ | ❏ | ❏ |
| 34. Toma cosas que no le pertenecen | ❏ | ❏ | ❏ |
| 35. Se rehusa a compartir | ❏ | ❏ | ❏ |

**Total**_____

Necesita usted ayuda con problemas de comportamiento, emocionales o aprendizaje?
____Si ____ No

# The Child Behavior Checklist (CBCL)
## (T. Achenbach & C.S. Edelbrock)

## Description

The Child Behavior Checklist (CBCL) is a tool on which parents or other individuals rate a child's problem behaviors and competencies. This Likert-Scale tool can either be self-administered or administered through an interview and now includes DSM-oriented scales. The CBCL also can be used to measure a child's change in behavior over time or following a treatment. The first section of the CBCL consists of 20 competence items and the second section consists of 120 items on behavior or emotional problems during the past 6 months (e.g., aggression, hyperactivity, bullying, conduct problems, defiance, and violence). Parents rate their child for how true each item is now or within the past 6 months using the following scale: 0 = not true (as far as you know); 1 = somewhat or sometimes true; and 2 = very true or often true. Teacher Report Forms (TRF), Youth Report Forms (YRF), and Direct Observation Forms are also available. It is suggested that the CBCL be used for further evaluation if a positive score is found on the Pediatric Symptom Checklist (PSC).

**Age Range:** Two versions of the tool exist: one for children 1 to 5 years of age and another for ages 6 to 18. The Youth Self Report tool is targeted for teens 11 to 18 years of age.

## Psychometric Properties of the CBCL

The CBCL has been extensively studied and supported by multiple studies to be a valid and highly reliable tool for use with African-American, Caucasian, and Hispanic/Latino children across all socioeconomic levels. The range of internal consistency reliability is reported as 0.78 to 0.97.

Manual and computer scoring is available.

Examiner Qualifications: Master's degree

**Permission Required to Use Instrument:** Yes

## Contact Information for Ordering the CBCL

Achenbach System of Empirically Based Assessment
1 South Prospect Street, Room 6436
Burlington, Vermont 05401-3456
Phone: 802-656-8313
Fax: 802-656-2608
Email: mail@aseba.org
Website: www.ASEBA.org

**Sources:** Achenbach, T. (1991). Integrative guide to the 1991 CBCL/4-18, YSR, and TRF Profiles. Burlington, VT: University of Vermont, Department of Psychology.
Achenbach, T. &  Edelbrock, C.S. (1983).  Manual for the Child Behavior Checklist and Revised Child Behavior Profile.  Burlington, VT: University of Vermont.

# Guidelines for Adolescent Preventive Services

Several tools have been designed to support implementing the American Medical Association's (AMA) Guidelines for Adolescent Preventive Services (GAPS) program in your clinical setting. The 6 forms that follow include the Younger Adolescent Questionnaire in English and Spanish, Middle-Older Adolescent Questionnaire in English and Spanish, and the Parent/Guardian Questionnaire in English and Spanish. The questionnaires are considered master copies that you can reproduce for use in clinical practice, but not alter, modify, or revise without the expressed written consent of the Child and Adolescent Health Program at the American Medical Association.

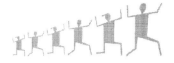

## Guidelines for Adolescent Preventive Services
### Younger Adolescent Questionnaire

**Confidential**  (Your answers will not be given out.)

Chart# _____

Name_____  Today's Date_____
        Last                        First              Middle Initial                          month    day    year

Birthdate _____  Grade in School _____   **Boy** or **Girl** (*circle one*)   Age _____
        month     day     year

Address_____  City_____State_____Zip_____

Phone Number_____  Pager/Beeper Number_____
            area code

What languages are spoken where you live? _____

Are you:     ☐ White                    ☐ African-American              ☐ Asian/Pacific Islander
             ☐ Latino/Hispanic          ☐ Native American              ☐ Other _____

### Medical History

1. Why did you come to the clinic/office today?_____

_____

2. Are you allergic to any medicines?
   ☐ No   ☐ Yes, name of medicine(s): _____   ☐ Not Sure

3. Do you have any health problems?
   ☐ No   ☐ Yes, problem(s): _____   ☐ Not Sure

4. Are you taking any medicine now?
   ☐ No   ☐ Yes, name of medicine(s): _____   ☐ Not Sure

5. Have you been to the dentist in the last year? ........................................................ ☐ No   ☐ Yes   ☐ Not Sure

6. Have you stayed overnight in a hospital in the last year?................................ ☐ No   ☐ Yes   ☐ Not Sure

7. Have you ever had any of the problems below?

|                        | Yes | No | Not Sure |           | Yes | No | Not Sure |
|------------------------|-----|----|----------|-----------|-----|----|----------|
| Allergies or hay fever | ☐   | ☐  | ☐        | Seizures  | ☐   | ☐  | ☐        |
| Asthma                 | ☐   | ☐  | ☐        | Cancer    | ☐   | ☐  | ☐        |
| Tuberculosis (TB)      | ☐   | ☐  | ☐        | Diabetes  | ☐   | ☐  | ☐        |

**For Girls Only**

8. Have you started having periods? .................................................................................. ☐ No  ☐ Yes

    a. *If yes*, are your periods regular (once a month) ? ................................................. ☐ No  ☐ Yes

    b. *If yes*, what was the 1st day of your last period?  Month _____ Day _____

9. Have you ever been pregnant? ...................................................................................... ☐ Yes  ☐ No

**Family Information**

10. Who do you live with?  (Check all that apply).

    ☐ Mother           ☐ Stepmother         ☐ Brother(s)/ages_____

    ☐ Father             ☐ Stepfather          ☐ Sister(s)/ages_____

    ☐ Guardian        ☐ Other adult relative    ☐ Other/(explain)_____

11. Do you have older brothers or sisters who live away from home? ........................... ☐ Yes  ☐ No  ☐ Not Sure

12. During the past year, have there been any changes in your family such as:  (Check all that apply)

    ☐ Marriage        ☐ Loss of job                ☐ Births              ☐ Other changes_____

    ☐ Separation    ☐ Moved to a new neighborhood    ☐ Serious Illness/Injury    _____

    ☐ Divorce        ☐ A new school               ☐ Deaths              _____

**Specific Health Issues**

13. Please check whether you have questions or are worried about any of the following:

    ☐ Height                ☐ Neck or back         ☐ Muscle or pain in arms/legs    ☐ Anger or temper

    ☐ Weight               ☐ Breasts              ☐ Menstruation or periods       ☐ Feeling tired

    ☐ Eyes or vision         ☐ Heart                 ☐ Wetting the bed            ☐ Trouble sleeping

    ☐ Hearing or earaches    ☐ Coughing or wheezing    ☐ Trouble urinating or peeing    ☐ Fitting in/belonging

    ☐ Colds/runny or         ☐ Chest pain or             ☐ Drip from penis or vagina    ☐ Cancer

        stuffy nose             trouble breathing

    ☐ Mouth or teeth or breath  ☐ Stomach ache        ☐ Wet dreams            ☐ HIV/AIDS

    ☐ Headaches           ☐ Vomiting or throwing up    ☐ Skin (rash/acne)       ☐ Dying

    ☐ Other_____

These questions will help us get to know you better. Choose the answer that best describes what you feel or do. Your answers will be seen only by your health care provider and his/her assistant.

**Health Profile**

**Eating/Weight/Body**

14. Do you eat fruits and vegetables every day? ................................................................ ☐ No  ☐ Yes

15. Do you drink milk and/or eat milk products every day? .......................................... ☐ No  ☐ Yes

16. Do you spend a lot of time thinking about ways to be skinny? ................................ ☐ Yes  ☐ No

17. Do you do things to lose weight (skip meals, take pills, starve yourself, vomit, etc) ........... ☐ Yes  ☐ No

18. Do you work, play, or exercise enough to make you sweat or breathe hard at least 3

    times a week? ................................................................................................................ ☐ No  ☐ Yes

19. Have you pierced your body (not including ears) or gotten a tattoo? ....................... ☐ Yes  ☐ No

## School

20. Is doing well in school important to you? ..................................................... ☐ No ☐ Yes
21. Is doing well in school important to your family and friends? ............................ ☐ No ☐ Yes
22. Are your grades this year worse than last year? ............................................ ☐ Yes ☐ No ☐ Not Sure
23. Are you getting failing grades in any subjects this year? ................................ ☐ Yes ☐ No ☐ Not Sure
24. Have you been told that you have a learning problem? .................................. ☐ Yes ☐ No
25. Have you been suspended from school this year? ......................................... ☐ Yes ☐ No

## Friends and Family

26. Do you know at least one person who you can talk to about problems? ............. ☐ No ☐ Yes
27. Do you think that your parent(s) or guardian(s) usually listen to you and take your feelings seriously? ................................................................... ☐ No ☐ Yes
28. Have your parents talked with you about things like alcohol, drugs, and sex? ..... ☐ No ☐ Yes ☐ Not Sure
29. Are you worried about problems at home or in your family? ........................... ☐ Yes ☐ No ☐ Not Sure
30. Have you ever thought seriously about running away from home? .................. ☐ Yes ☐ No

## Weapons/Violence/Safety

31. Is there a gun, rifle, or other firearm where you live? .................................. ☐ Yes ☐ No ☐ Not Sure
32. Have you ever carried a gun, knife, club, or other weapon to protect yourself? ... ☐ Yes ☐ No
33. Have you ever been in a physical fight where you or someone else got hurt? ...... ☐ Yes ☐ No
34. Have you ever been in trouble with the police? .......................................... ☐ Yes ☐ No
35. Have you ever seen a violent act take place at home, school, or in your neighborhood? .... ☐ Yes ☐ No
36. Are you worried about violence or your safety? .......................................... ☐ Yes ☐ No ☐ Not Sure
37. Do you usually wear a helmet and/or protective gear when you rollerblade, skateboard, or ride a bike? ................................................................... ☐ No ☐ Yes
38. Do you always wear a seat belt when you ride in a car, truck, or van? .............. ☐ No ☐ Yes

## Tobacco

39. Have you ever tried cigarettes or chewing tobacco? .................................... ☐ Yes ☐ No
40. Have any of your close friends ever tried cigarettes or chewing tobacco? ......... ☐ Yes ☐ No
41. Does anyone you live with smoke cigarettes/cigars or chew tobacco? ............. ☐ Yes ☐ No

## Alcohol

42. Have you ever tried beer, wine, or other liquor (except for religious purposes)? .. ☐ Yes ☐ No
43. Have any of your close friends ever tried beer, wine, or other liquor (except for religious purposes)? ................................................................. ☐ Yes ☐ No
44. Have you ever been in a car when the driver has been using drugs or drinking beer, wine or other liquor? ....................................................................... ☐ Yes ☐ No
45. Does anyone in your family drink so much that it worries you? ....................... ☐ Yes ☐ No ☐ Not Sure

## Drugs

46. Have you ever taken things to get high, stay awake, calm down or go to sleep? ... ☐ Yes ☐ No ☐ Not Sure
47. Have you ever used marijuana (pot, grass, weed, reefer, or blunt)? ................. ☐ Yes ☐ No ☐ Not Sure
48. Have you ever used other drugs such as cocaine, speed, LSD, mushrooms, etc.? ... ☐ Yes ☐ No ☐ Not Sure
49. Have you ever sniffed or huffed things like paint, 'white-out', glue, gasoline, etc.? ... ☐ Yes ☐ No ☐ Not Sure

50. Have any of your close friends ever used marijuana, other drugs, or done other things to get high? ................................................................................ ☐ Yes ☐ No ☐ Not Sure

51. Does anyone in your family use drugs so much that it worries you? ....................................... ☐ Yes ☐ No ☐ Not Sure

## Development/Relationships

52. Are you dating someone or going steady? ............................................................................ ☐ Yes ☐ No ☐ Not Sure

53. Are you thinking about having sex ("going all the way "or "doing it")? ................................. ☐ Yes ☐ No ☐ Not Sure

54. Have you ever had sex? ............................................................................................................ ☐ Yes ☐ No ☐ Not Sure

55. Have any of your friends ever had sex? .................................................................................. ☐ Yes ☐ No ☐ Not Sure

56. Have you ever felt pressured by anyone to have sex or had sex when you did not want to? .......... ☐ Yes ☐ No ☐ Not Sure

57. Have you ever been told by a doctor or a nurse that you had a sexually transmitted disease like herpes, gonorrhea, or chlamydia? ................................................................... ☐ Yes ☐ No ☐ Not Sure

58. Would you like to receive information on abstinence ("how to say no to sex")? ................... ☐ Yes ☐ No ☐ Not Sure

59. Would you like to know how to avoid getting pregnant, getting HIV/AIDS, or getting sexually transmitted diseases? ............................................................................................ ☐ Yes ☐ No ☐ Not Sure

## Emotions

60. Have you done something fun during the past two weeks? ................................................. ☐ No ☐ Yes

61. When you get angry, do you do violent things? ................................................................... ☐ Yes ☐ No

62. During the past few weeks, have you felt very sad or down as though you have nothing to look forward to? ................................................................................................. ☐ Yes ☐ No

63. Have you ever seriously thought about killing yourself, made a plan, or tried to kill yourself? .......... ☐ Yes ☐ No

64. Is there something you often worry about or fear? ............................................................. ☐ Yes ☐ No

65. Have you ever been physically, emotionally, or sexually abused? ...................................... ☐ Yes ☐ No ☐ Not Sure

66. Would you like to get counseling about something that is bothering you? ........................... ☐ Yes ☐ No ☐ Not Sure

## Special Circumstances

67. In the past year have you been around someone with tuberculosis (TB)? ........................... ☐ Yes ☐ No ☐ Not Sure

68. In the past year, have you stayed overnight in a homeless shelter, jail, or detention center? ............. ☐ Yes ☐ No

69. Have you ever lived in foster care or a group home? ........................................................... ☐ Yes ☐ No

## Self

70. What two words best describe you?

1)_____ 2)_____

71. What would you like to be when you grow up?

_____

72. If you could have three wishes come true, what would they be?

1)_____

2)_____

3)_____

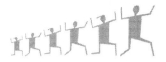

Archivo #_____

Nombre_____Fecha de Hoy _____
     (Apellido)                (Nombre)             (Inicial)          mes/día/año

Fecha de Nacimiento_____ Año/Curso Escolar_____ Niño o Niña *(marque con círculo)* Edad_____
             mes/día/año

Dirección_____ Ciudad_____ Código Postal/Zip_____

Teléfono ( )_____ Anunciador/Pager/Beeper ( )_____
     Código

¿ Cuales idiomas se hablan donde vive Ud.? _____

¿Es Ud.?:      ☐ Blanco      ☐ Afro-Americano      ☐ Asiático/Isleño del Pacífico
                ☐ Latino/Hispano      ☐ Indígena Norteamericano      ☐ Otro

## Historia Médica

1. ¿Porqué vino al consultorio hoy?_____

_____

2. ¿Tiene alergias a cualquier medicina?
   ☐ No     ☐ Sí, (nombre(s) de la(s) medicina(s):_____ )  ☐ No estoy seguro

3. ¿Tiene cualquier problema con la salud?
   ☐ No     ☐ Sí, (problema(s): _____)  ☐ No estoy seguro

4. ¿Esta tomando medicinas actualmente?
   ☐ No     ☐ Sí, (nombre de la medicina(s):_____)  ☐ No estoy seguro

5. ¿En el último año ha consultado al dentista?........................................ ☐ No  ☐ Sí  ☐ No estoy seguro

6. En el último año Ha pasado la noche en el hospital?........................ ☐ No  ☐ Sí  ☐ No estoy seguro

7. ¿Alguna vez padeció cualquiera de los siguientes problemas de salud?

|  | Sí | No | No estoy seguro |  | Sí | No | No estoy seguro |
|---|---|---|---|---|---|---|---|
| Alergias o "hay fever" | ☐ | ☐ | ☐ | Convulsiones/Ataques | ☐ | ☐ | ☐ |
| Asma | ☐ | ☐ | ☐ | Cáncer | ☐ | ☐ | ☐ |
| Tuberculosis (TB) | ☐ | ☐ | ☑ | Diabetes | ☐ | ☐ | ☐ |

## Unicamente para Niñas

8. Ha comenzado a tener su período/ la regla? ........................................☐ No ☐ Sí

   a. Si ya comenzó Le viene regularmente (una vez al mes)?...................☐ No ☐ Sí

   b. Si es el caso, ¿Cual fue el primer día de la última regla?...................Mes ____ Día____

9. ¿Alguna vez ha estado embarazada? ....................................................☐ No ☐ Sí

## Información Familiar

10. ¿Con quién vive? (Marque todas que sean ciertas).

- [ ] Madre
- [ ] Padre
- [ ] Guardián Legal

- [ ] Madrastra
- [ ] Padrastro
- [ ] Otro pariente adulto

- [ ] Hermanos/edades
- [ ] Hermanas/edades
- [ ] Otra/(explique)

11. ¿Tiene hermanos mayores que no viven en casa?.................................................. [ ] Sí  [ ] No      [ ] No estoy seguro

12. En el último año Han habido cambios importantes en su familia? (Marque todas que sean ciertas),

- [ ] Matrimonios
- [ ] Separaciones
- [ ] Divorcios

- [ ] Alguien perdi su empleo
- [ ] Mudanzas a otros vecindarios
- [ ] Cambio de escuela

- [ ] Nacimientos
- [ ] Enfermedades graves
- [ ] Muertes

- [ ] Otros cambios

## Problemas Específicos de la Salud

13. Por favor, marque a continuación si tiene preguntas o alguna preocupación sobre:

- [ ] Estatura/desarrollo físico
- [ ] Peso
- [ ] Ojos/la vista
- [ ] Dificultad para oir o dolor del oído
- [ ] Catarro/moquillo o las narices tapadas
- [ ] Boca o dientes o aliento
- [ ] Dolores de cabeza
- [ ] Otro _____

- [ ] Cuello o espalda
- [ ] Pechos/senos
- [ ] Corazón
- [ ] Tos o le chilla el pecho  hacer pipí
- [ ] Dolor del pecho o dificultad en respirar
- [ ] Dolor del estómago
- [ ] Vómito o náuseas

- [ ] Músculos o dolor en los brazos/piernas
- [ ] Menstruación o la regla
- [ ] Mojarse la cama
- [ ] Dificultad para orinar o
- [ ] Gota del pene o la vagina
- [ ] Sueño mojado
- [ ] Piel (salpullido/espinillas)

- [ ] Enojo o mal genio
- [ ] Cansancio
- [ ] Dificultad al dormir
- [ ] Su relación con los compañeros
- [ ] Cáncer
- [ ] VIH/SIDA
- [ ] La muerte

Estas preguntas nos ayudarán a conocerle mejor. Escoja la respuesta que mejor indica lo que siente o hace.
Sus respuestas ser n vistas nicamente por su médico/enfermera y su asistente.

## Su Salud

Comer/Peso/Cuerpo

14. ¿Come Ud. frutas y vegetales cada día? .................................................[ ] No  [ ] Sí

15. ¿Toma Ud. leche y/o come productos lácteos cada día? .........................[ ] No  [ ] Sí

16. ¿Gasta mucho tiempo pensando en como adelgazar? ............................[ ] Sí  [ ] No

17. ¿Trata de bajar de peso (evita comidas, toma pastillas, ayuna, vomita, eta) .....[ ] Sí  [ ] No

18. ¿Trabaja Ud, juega, o hace suficiente ejercicio como para sudar o respirar fuerte por lo menos 3 veces por semana? ................................[ ] No [ ] Sí

19. Ha perforado su cuerpo (sin incluir las orejas) o ha puesto un tatuaje? ...........[ ] Sí  [ ] No

**La Escuela**

20. ¿Salir bien en sus estudios es importante para Ud.? .............................[ ] No  [ ] Sí

21. ¿Salir bien en sus estudios es importante para su familia y sus amigos?...........[ ] No  [ ] Sí

22. ¿Sus notas (calificaciones) son peores este año ? ..................................[ ] Sí  [ ] No      [ ] No estoy seguro

23. ¿Está saliendo mal en alguna materia ? .................................................[ ] Sí  [ ] No      [ ] No estoy seguro

24. ¿Le han dicho que tiene dificultad en aprender? .....................................[ ] Sí  [ ] No

25. ¿Le han suspendido de clases este año?.................................................[ ] Sí  [ ] No

## Los Amigos y la Familia

26. ¿Conoce al menos una persona con quien puede hablar si tiene un problema? ☐ No ☐ Sí
27. ¿ Cree Ud. que sus padres o su guardián le
    escuchan y toman en serio sus sentimientos? ........................................☐ No ☐ Sí
28. ¿Sus padres han hablado con Ud. sobre alcohol, drogas, y sexo ? ......☐ No ☐ Sí        ☐ No estoy seguro
29. ¿Está preocupado por problemas en su casa o en su familia ? ............☐ Sí ☐ No        ☐ No estoy seguro
30. ¿Alguna vez ha contemplado seriamente fugarse de la casa? ..............☐ Sí ☐ No

## Las Armas/la Violencia/la Seguridad

31. ¿Hay una pistola, rifle u otra arma de fuego en la casa donde vive ? ................☐ Sí ☐ No        ☐ No estoy seguro
32. ¿Alguna vez ha portado una pistola, cuchillo,
    palo u otra arma para protegerse? ..............................................☐ Sí ☐ No
33. ¿Alguna vez ha estado en una pelea donde Ud. u otra persona fue lesionado? ..☐ Sí ☐ No
34. ¿Alguna vez ha tenido problemas con la policía? ........................☐ Sí ☐ No
35. ¿Alguna vez ha visto un acto de violencia en la casa, la escuela,
    o en el vecindario? ..........................................................☐ Sí ☐ No
36. ¿Está Ud. preocupado por la violencia o por su seguridad? ................☐ Sí ☐ No        ☐ No estoy seguro
37. ¿Normalmente usa Ud. un casco y/o equipo protectivo cuando patina
    ("roller blade," "skateboard", o monta a bicicleta)? ......................☐ No ☐ Sí
38. ¿Siempre usa Ud. el cinturón de seguridad cuando monta
    en un auto, vehículo de carga, o camioneta? ..............................☐ No ☐ Sí

## El Tabaco

39. Ha probado Ud. cigarrillos o tabaco de mascar (rapé)? ................☐ Sí ☐ No
40. ¿Alguno de sus mejores amigos ha probado cigarrillos o tabaco de mascar? ......☐ Sí ☐ No
41. ¿Alguien con quien vive Ud. fuma cigarrillos/puros o usa tabaco de mascar? ....☐ Sí ☐ No

## El Alcohol

42. ¿Alguna vez ha probado Ud. cerveza, vino, u otro licor
    (fuera de propósitos religiosos)? ..........................................☐ Sí ☐ No
43. ¿Alguno de sus mejores amigos ha probado cerveza, vino, u otro licor
    (fuera de propósitos religiosos)? ..........................................☐ Sí ☐ No
44. ¿Alguna vez ha estado en un veh culo cuando el motorista ha estado
    tomando drogas, cerveza, vino, u otro licor? ..............................☐ Sí ☐ No
45. ¿Hay alguien en su familia que toma tanto que le preocupa? ..............☐ Sí ☐ No        ☐ No estoy seguro

## Las Drogas

46. ¿Alguna vez ha tomado sustancias para elevarse, para
    mantenerse despierto, calmarse, o para dormir? ..........................☐ Sí ☐ No        ☐ No estoy seguro
47. ¿Alguna vez ha usado marijuana
    (hierba, pasto, maría, mota, "refer, o pot")? ..............................☐ Sí ☐ No        ☐ No estoy seguro
48. ¿Alguna vez ha usado otras drogas como la coca na,
    la metanfetamina "speed", LSD, hongos.? ................................☐ Sí ☐ No        ☐ No estoy seguro
49. ¿Alguna vez ha inhalado sustancias: pintura, "white-out",
    gases de los pegantes o gomas, gasolina? ................................☐ Sí ☐ No        ☐ No estoy seguro
50. ¿Alguno de sus mejores amigos ha usado la marijuana, otras drogas o
    hecho otras cosas para elevarse o sentirse "bien"? ......................☐ Sí ☐ No        ☐ No estoy seguro
51. ¿Hay alguien en su familia que usa tanta droga que le preocupa? ......☐ Sí ☐ No        ☐ No estoy seguro

## El Desarrollo/Relaciones Personales

52. ¿Tiene novio(a) o esta saliendo con alguien?.................................☐ Sí  ☐ No  ☐ No estoy seguro
53. ¿Está pensando en tener relaciones sexuales (en hacerlo, tener sexo)?...........☐ Sí  ☐ No  ☐ No estoy seguro
54. ¿Quisiera recibir información sobre como abstenerse
    (como decir que "no" a tener sexo)?..........................................☐ Sí  ☐ No  ☐ No estoy seguro
55. ¿Alguna vez ha tenido relaciones sexuales?.....................................☐ Sí  ☐ No  ☐ No estoy seguro
56. ¿Alguno de sus amigos ha tenido relaciones sexuales ya?........................☐ Sí  ☐ No  ☐ No estoy seguro
57. ¿Alguna vez ha sido presionado por alguien a tener
    relaciones o ha tenido relaciones cuando no quería? ......................☐ Sí  ☐ No  ☐ No estoy seguro
58. ¿Alguna vez un médico le ha dicho que tuvo una enfermedad
    transmitida sexualmente como el herpes, la gonorrea, o la sífilis?.......☐ Sí  ☐ No  ☐ No estoy seguro
59. ¿Quisiera saber como evitar el embarazo, el VIH/SIDA,
    o una enfermedad "venérea"?...............................................☐ Sí  ☐ No  ☐ No estoy seguro

## Las Emociones

60. ¿ Ha hecho algo divertido en las últimas dos semanas? ......................☐ No  ☐ Sí
61. ¿Cuando se pone enojado, se hace cosas violentas?..........................☐ No  ☐ Sí
62. ¿Durante las últimas semanas ha sentido muy triste,
    desanimado, desalentado? ................................................☐ No  ☐ Sí
63. ¿Alguna vez ha pensado seriamente en matarse,
    ha hecho un plan, o ha intentado matarse? ..............................☐ No  ☐ Sí
64. ¿Hay algo que le preocupa o teme con frecuencia?..........................☐ No  ☐ Sí
65. ¿Alguna vez ha sido abusado físicamente, emocionalmente, o sexualmente? ....☐ No  ☐ Sí  ☐ No estoy seguro
66. ¿Quisiera hablar con un(a) consejero(a) de algo que le preocupa? .................☐ No  ☐ Sí  ☐ No estoy seguro

## Circunstancias Especiales

67. En este año pasado, ¿Ha pasado tiempo con alguien
    que tiene la tuberculosis?................................................☐ Sí  ☐ No  ☐ No estoy seguro
68. En este año pasado, ¿Ha pasado la noche en un albergue,
    la cárcel, o un centro detención juvenil? ...............................☐ Sí  ☐ No
69. ¿Alguna vez ha vivido con padres de crianza, o en una casa juvenil?.................☐ Sí  ☐ No

## Sí Mismo

70. ¿Cuales dos palabras describen mejor a Ud.?  1)_____  2)_____

71. ¿Que quiere hacer cuando sea adulto?_____
72. Si podrían concederle tres deseos, cuales serían?

    1)_____

    2)_____

    3)_____

Febrero, 1998

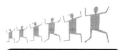

**Confidential** (Your answers will not be given out.)                    Chart # _____

Name _____ Date _____
         Last                          First                          Middle Initial

Date of Birth _____ Grade in School_____ Year in college_____ Sex: Male Female Age _____

Address _____ City _____ Zip _____

Phone number where you can be reached _____ Pager/beeper number_____

What languages are spoken where you live? _____ Race _____

## Medical History

1. Why did you come to the clinic/office today? _____

2. Do you have any health problems? ☐ Yes ☐ No  Problem(s) _____

3. Did you have any health problems in the past 12 months? ☐ Yes ☐ No  Problem(s) _____

4. Are you taking any medicine now? ☐ Yes ☐ No  Name of medicine _____

### For Girls

5. Date when last period started_____ Are your periods regular (monthly)? . . . . . . . . . . . ☐ No   ☐ Yes
                                    Month         Date

6. Have you had a miscarriage, an abortion, or live birth in the past 12 months? . . . . . . . . . . . . . . . . . . . . . . . . . . . . . . ☐ Yes   ☐ No

## Specific Health Issues

7. Please check whether you have questions or are worried about any of the following:

| | | | |
|---|---|---|---|
| ☐ Height/weight | ☐ Mouth/teeth/breath | ☐ Frequent or painful urination | ☐ Trouble sleeping |
| ☐ Blood pressure | ☐ Neck/back | | ☐ Feeling tired a lot |
| ☐ Diet/food/appetite | ☐ Chest pain/trouble breathing | ☐ Discharge from penis or vagina | ☐ Cancer |
| ☐ Future plans/job | | ☐ Wetting the bed | ☐ Dying |
| ☐ Skin (rash, acne) | ☐ Coughing/wheezing | ☐ Sexual organs/genitals | ☐ Sad or crying a lot |
| ☐ Headaches/migraines | ☐ Breasts | ☐ Menstruation/periods | ☐ Stress |
| ☐ Dizziness/fainting | ☐ Heart | ☐ Wet dreams | ☐ Anger/temper |
| ☐ Eyes/vision | ☐ Stomach ache | ☐ Physical or sexual abuse | ☐ Violence/personal safety |
| ☐ Ears/hearing/ear aches | ☐ Nausea/vomiting | ☐ Masturbation | ☐ Other (explain) |
| ☐ Nose | ☐ Diarrhea/constipation | ☐ HIV/AIDS | _____ |
| ☐ Lots of colds | ☐ Muscle or joint pain in arms/legs | | _____ |

## Health Profile

These questions will help us get to know you better. Choose the answer that best describes what you feel or do. Your answers will be seen only by your health care provider and his/her assistant.

### Eating/Weight

8. Are you satisfied with your eating habits?. . . . . . . . . . . . . . . . . . . . . . . . . . . . . . . . . . . . . . . . ☐ No     ☐ Yes

9. Do you ever eat in secret? . . . . . . . . . . . . . . . . . . . . . . . . . . . . . . . . . . . . . . . . . . . . . . . . . . ☐ Yes    ☐ No

10. Do you spend a lot of time thinking about ways to be thin? . . . . . . . . . . . . . . . . . . . . . . . . . . . . . ☐ Yes    ☐ No

11. In the past year, have you tried to lose weight or control your weight by vomiting, taking diet pills or laxatives, or starving yourself?. . . . . . . . . . . . . . . . . . . . . . . . . . . . . . . . ☐ Yes    ☐ No

12. Do you exercise or participate in sport activities that make you sweat and breathe hard for 20 minutes or more at a time at least three or more times during the week?. . . . . . . . . . . . . . . ☐ No     ☐ Yes

### School

13. Are your grades this year worse than last year? . . . . . . . . . . . . . . . . . . . . . . . . . . . . . . . . . . . . ☐ Yes    ☐ No    ☐ Not in school

14. Have you either been told you have a learning problem or do you think you have a learning problem? . . . . . . . . . . . ☐ Yes    ☐ No

15. Have you been suspended from school this year?. . . . . . . . . . . . . . . . . . . . . . . . . . . . . . . . . . . ☐ Yes    ☐ No    ☐ Not in school

### Friends & Family

16. Do you have at least one friend who you really like and feel you can talk to?. . . . . . . . . . . . . . . . . . . . . . ☐ No     ☐ Yes

17. Do you think that your parent(s) or guardian(s) *usually* listen to you and take your feelings seriously? . . . . . . ☐ No     ☐ Yes

18. Have you ever thought seriously about running away from home?. . . . . . . . . . . . . . . . . . . . . . . . . . . . ☐ Yes    ☐ No    ☐ Not sure

**Turn page**

**Weapons/Violence/Safety**

19. Do you or anyone you live with have a gun, rifle, or other firearm? .................................... ☐ Yes ☐ No ☐ Not sure

20. In the past year, have you carried a gun, knife, club, or other weapon for protection? ..................... ☐ Yes ☐ No

21. Have you been in a physical fight during the *past 3 months*? ......................................... ☐ Yes ☐ No

22. Have you ever been in trouble with the law? ....................................................... ☐ Yes ☐ No

23. Are you worried about violence or your safety? .................................................... ☐ Yes ☐ No ☐ Not sure

24. Do you usually wear a helmet when you rollerblade, skateboard, ride a bicycle, motorcycle, minibike, or ride in an all-terrain vehicle (ATV)? ........................................... ☐ No ☐ Yes

25. Do you usually wear a seat belt when you ride in or drive a car, truck, or van? ........................ ☐ No ☐ Yes

**Tobacco**

26. Do you ever smoke cigarettes/cigars, use snuff or chew tobacco? ....................................... ☐ Yes ☐ No

26. Do any of your close friends ever smoke cigarettes/cigars, use snuff or chew tobacco? ..................... ☐ Yes ☐ No

28. Does anyone you live with smoke cigarettes/cigars, use snuff or chew tobacco? ........................... ☐ Yes ☐ No

**Alcohol**

29. In the past month, did you get drunk or very high on beer, wine, or other alcohol? ..................... ☐ Yes ☐ No

30. In the past month, did any of your close friends get drunk or very high on beer, wine, or other alcohol? .......... ☐ Yes ☐ No

31. Have you ever been criticized or gotten into trouble because of drinking? ............................. ☐ Yes ☐ No ☐ Not sure

32. In the past year have you used alcohol and then driven a car/truck/van/motorcycle? ..................... ☐ Yes ☐ No ☐ Does not apply

33. In the past year, have you been in a car or other motor vehicle when the driver has been drinking alcohol or using drugs? ............................................... ☐ Yes ☐ No

34. Does anyone in your family drink or take drugs so much that it worries you? ........................... ☐ Yes ☐ No

**Drugs**

35. Do you ever use marijuana or other drugs, or sniff inhalants? ....................................... ☐ Yes ☐ No ☐ Not sure

36. Do any of your close friends ever use marijuana or other drugs, or sniff inhalants? ..................... ☐ Yes ☐ No ☐ Not sure

37. Do you ever use non-prescription drugs to get to sleep, stay awake, calm down, or get high? (These drugs can be bought at a store without a doctor's prescription.) ................................... ☐ Yes ☐ No

38. Have you ever used steroid pills or shots without a doctor telling you to? ............................. ☐ Yes ☐ No ☐ Not sure

**Development**

39. Do you have any concerns or questions about the size or shape of your body, or your physical appearance? ............................................................... ☐ Yes ☐ No ☐ Not sure

40. Do you think you may be gay, lesbian, or bisexual? ................................................ ☐ Yes ☐ No ☐ Not sure

41. Have you ever had sexual intercourse? (How old were you the first time?_____) ............ ☐ Yes ☐ No ☐ Not sure

42. Are you using a method to prevent pregnancy? (Which:_____) .......... ☐ No ☐ Yes ☐ Not active

43. Do you and your partner(s) *always* use condoms when you have sex? ................................ ☐ No ☐ Yes ☐ Not active

44. Have any of your close friends ever had sexual intercourse? ......................................... ☐ Yes ☐ No ☐ Not sure

45. Have you ever been told by a doctor or nurse that you had a sexually transmitted infection or disease? ....... ☐ Yes ☐ No ☐ Not sure

46. Have you ever been pregnant or gotten someone pregnant? ........................................... ☐ Yes ☐ No ☐ Not sure

47. Would you like to receive information or supplies to prevent pregnancy or sexually transmitted infections? ... ☐ Yes ☐ No ☐ Not sure

48. Would you like to know how to avoid getting HIV/AIDS? ............................................. ☐ Yes ☐ No ☐ Not sure

49. Have you pierced your body (not including ears) or gotten a tattoo? ................................... ☐ Yes ☐ No ☐ Thinking about it

**Emotions**

50. Have you had fun during the past two weeks? ...................................................... ☐ No ☐ Yes

51. During the past few weeks, have you *often* felt sad or down or as though you have nothing to look forward to? ........................................................... ☐ Yes ☐ No

52. Have you ever *seriously* thought about killing yourself, made a plan or actually tried to kill yourself? ........ ☐ Yes ☐ No

53. Have you ever been physically, sexually, or emotionally abused? ...................................... ☐ Yes ☐ No ☐ Not sure

54. When you get angry, do you do violent things? .................................................... ☐ Yes ☐ No

55. Would you like to get counseling about something you have on your mind? ............................... ☐ Yes ☐ No ☐ Not sure

**Special Circumstances**

56. In the past year, have you been around someone with tuberculosis (TB)? ............................... ☐ Yes ☐ No ☐ Not sure
57. In the past year, have you stayed overnight in a homeless shelter, jail, or detention center? ............... ☐ Yes ☐ No
58. Have you ever lived in foster care or a group home? ................................................ ☐ Yes ☐ No

**Self**

59. What four words best describe you? _____

60. If you could change one thing about your life or yourself, what would it be? _____
_____

61. What do you want to talk about today? _____

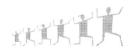

## Guía De Servicios Preventivos Adolescentes
## Cuestionario Mayores Para Adolescentes

**Confidencial** (No le diremos a nadie lo que tú nos digas)         Expediente # _____

Nombre_____ Fecha_____
             (apellido)              (nombre)              (inicial del segundo nombre)

Fecha de nacimiento _____Año Escolar _____Año Universitario _____Sexo: ❏ Hombre ❏ Mujer   Edad_____

Dirección_____Ciudad_____Area Postal_____

Teléfono donde te podemos llamar_____Beeper_____

¿Qué idiomas se hablan en tu hogar?_____Raza_____

### Historial Médico

1. ¿Por qué viniste hoy a la clínica/oficina? _____

2. ¿Tienes algún problema de salud? ❏ Sí ❏ No  Problema(s) _____

3. ¿Has tenido algún problema de salud en el año pasado?         ❏ Sí   ❏ No

4. ¿Estás tomando alguna medicina ahora? ❏ Sí ❏ No  Nombre de la medicina_____

### Para Mujeres Jóvenes

5. ¿Cuál fue el primer día de tu última regla? _____ ¿Te viene la regla regularmente cada mes? .................. ❏ No      ❏ Sí

6. ¿Has tenido un aborto (natural o provocado) o has tenido un hijo en los ultimos 12 meses? ......................... ❏ Sí      ❏ No

### Sobre La Salud

7. Si tienes alguna pregunta o preocupación sobre alguno de los siguientes temas, márcalos.

❏ Estatura/peso
❏ Alta o baja presión
❏ Dieta/comida/apetito
❏ Planes para el futuro/trabajo
❏ Piel (sarpullido, acné)
❏ Dolores de cabeza/migrañas
❏ Mareos/desmayos
❏ Ojos/visión
❏ Oídos/dolor de oídos
❏ Nariz
❏ Muchos catarros
❏ Boca/dientes/aliento
❏ Cuello/espalda
❏ Dolor de pecho/dificultad al respirar

❏ Tos/te silba el pecho
❏ Senos (el busto)
❏ Corazón
❏ Dolores de estómago
❏ Náusea/vómitos
❏ Diarrea/estreñimiento
❏ Dolor muscular o en las articulaciones
❏ Orinas frecuentemente o tienes dolor al orinar
❏ Secreción del pene o de la vagina
❏ Te orinas en la cama
❏ Organos sexuales/genitales
❏ Menstruación/regla

❏ Eyaculas cuando sueñas (el despertar mojado)
❏ Abuso físico o sexual
❏ Masturbación
❏ VIH/SIDA
❏ No duermes bien
❏ Cansancio todo el tiempo
❏ Cáncer
❏ La muerte
❏ Triste o lloras mucho
❏ Estrés
❏ Enojo/mal humor
❏ Violencia/seguridad personal

❏ Otros (explica) _____

### Tu Salud

Estas preguntas nos ayudarán a conocerte mejor.  Escoge la respuesta que mejor describe lo que sientes o haces. Tus respuestas sólo las repasan el doctor y su asistente.

#### Dieta/Peso

8. ¿Estás satisfecho con tus hábitos alimenticios?................................................❏ No  ❏ Sí

9. ¿Comes a escondidas o en secreto de vez en cuando? .....................................❏ Sí   ❏ No

10. ¿Te pasas horas pensando en cómo bajar de peso? ..........................................❏ Sí   ❏ No

11. En el año pasado, ¿trataste de bajar o controlar tu peso haciéndote vomitar, usando pastillas, laxantes o purgantes, o dejando de comer? .............................❏ Sí   ❏ No

12. ¿Haces ejercicios o participas en actividades deportivas tres veces o más durante la semana que te hacen sudar y respirar fuerte y que duran 20 minutos? ..........❏ No  ❏ Sí

                                      Voltee la página

## Escuela

13. ¿Tus notas de este año son peores que las del año pasado? ........................ ❏ Sí    ❏ No   ❏ No estoy en la escuela

14. ¿Te han dicho o piensas que tienes problemas para aprender? ..................... ❏ Sí    ❏ No

15. ¿Te han suspendido de clases en la escuela este año? ................................... ❏ Sí    ❏ No   ❏ No estoy en la escuela

## Amistades y Familia

16. ¿Tienes un amigo a quien estimas mucho y con quien puedes hablar de todo? ............ ❏ No    ❏ Sí

17. ¿Piensas que tus padres o tus guardianes te escuchan usualmente y te toman tus sentamientos en serio? ......................................................................... ❏ No    ❏ Sí

18. ¿Alguna vez has pensado seriamente en escaparte de tu casa? ...................... ❏ Sí    ❏ No   ❏ No estoy seguro(a)

## Armas/Violencia/Seguridad

19. ¿Alguna de las personas con quien vives tú mismo tiene una pistola, rifle, o alguna otra arma de fuego? ........................................................................ ❏ Sí    ❏ No   ❏ No estoy seguro(a)

20. ¿Has portado una pistola, navaja, garrote o alguna otra arma para protegerte en los últimos 12 meses? ....................................................................... ❏ Sí    ❏ No

21. ¿Has tenido alguna pelea física en los últimos 3 meses? ............................... ❏ Sí    ❏ No

22. ¿Has tenido problemas con la ley? ............................................................... ❏ Sí    ❏ No

23. ¿Te preocupa la violencia o tu seguridad? .................................................... ❏ Sí    ❏ No   ❏ No estoy seguro(a)

24. ¿Usas un casco cuando montas en patines, patineta, bicicleta, motocicleta, miniciclo, trimoto o arenero? ...................................................................... ❏ No    ❏ Sí

25. ¿Usas el cinturón de seguridad cuando viajas en carro, camión, o camioneta? ............. ❏ No    ❏ Sí

## Tabaco

26. ¿Fumas cigarrillos/puros, masticas tabaco, o usas "snuff?" ........................... ❏ Sí    ❏ No

27. ¿Alguno de tus amigos fuma cigarrillos/puros, mastica tabaco, o usa "snuff?" ............... ❏ Sí    ❏ No

28. ¿Alguna de las personas con quien vives fuma cigarrillos/puros, mastica tabaco, o usa "snuff?" ....................................................................................... ❏ Sí    ❏ No

## Alcohol

29. El mes pasado, ¿tuviste una borrachera con cerveza, vino, o alguna otra bebida alcohólica? ...................................................................................... ❏ Sí    ❏ No

30. El mes pasado, ¿alguno de tus mejores amigos tuvo una borrachera con cerveza, vino, o alguna otra bebida alcohólica? ......................................................... ❏ Sí    ❏ No

31. ¿Alguna vez te han criticado o has tenido problemas porque tomas? ........... ❏ Sí    ❏ No   ❏ No estoy seguro(a)

32. ¿Bebiste alcohol este año pasado, y después manejaste un carro, camión, camioneta o motocicleta? ......................................................................... ❏ Sí    ❏ No   ❏ No aplica

33. ¿Estuviste en un carro o algún otro vehículo este año pasado, en el cual el chofer estaba bebido o había usado drogas? .................................................... ❏ Sí    ❏ No

34. ¿Te preocupas por alguno de tu familia que toma mucho o usa drogas? ...................... ❏ Sí    ❏ No

## Drogas

35. ¿A veces usas marihuana u otras drogas, o inhalas goma o cosas parecidas? ................. ❏ Sí    ❏ No   ❏ No estoy seguro(a)

36. ¿Alguno de tus mejores amigos usa marihuana u otras drogas, o inhala goma o cosas parecidas? .................................................................................. ❏ Sí    ❏ No   ❏ No estoy seguro(a)

37. ¿Alguna vez has usado medicinas sin receta médica para poder dormir, estar despierto, calmarte, o ponerte en onda? .................................................. ❏ Sí    ❏ No
(Medicinas que se pueden comprar en cualquier farmacia, sin receta médica)

38. ¿Has usado esteroides en pastilla o como inyección sin receta medica? ......................... ❏ Sí    ❏ No   ❏ No estoy seguro(a)

## Desarrollo

39. ¿Te preocupa o quieres más información sobre la forma o tamaño de tu cuerpo, o tu apariencia física? ............................................................................... ❏ Sí    ❏ No   ❏ No estoy seguro(a)

40. ¿Crees ser homosexual, lesbiana, o bisexual? .............................................. ❏ Sí    ❏ No   ❏ No estoy seguro(a)

41. ¿Has tenido relaciones sexuales? ......................................................... ❑ Sí    ❑ No ❑ No estoy seguro(a)
    ¿Cuántos años tenías la primera vez?_____

42. ¿Estás usando algún método para prevenir el embarazo? ..................... ❑ No    ❑ Sí   ❑ No tengo relaciones
    ¿Cuál? _____

43. ¿Usas condones cuando siempre tienes relaciones sexuales con tus pareja(s)? ............ ❑ No    ❑ Sí   ❑ No tengo relaciones

44. ¿Alguno de tus mejores amigos ha tenido relaciones sexuales? ............... ❑ Sí    ❑ No ❑ No estoy seguro(a)

45. ¿Te ha dicho alguna vez algún doctor o enfermera que tienes una enfermedad o infección que se transmite sexualmente? ........................................... ❑ Sí    ❑ No ❑ No estoy seguro(a)

46. ¿Has estado embarazada alguna vez, o has sido tú el que embarazó a alguna joven? .. ❑ Sí    ❑ No ❑ No estoy seguro(a)

47. ¿Quieres información o cosas que te ayuden a evitar embarazos, o infecciones transmitidas sexualmente? ................................................................. ❑ Sí    ❑ No ❑ No estoy seguro(a)

48. ¿Quieres saber cómo evitar contraer el virus del VIH/SIDA? ............................. ❑ Sí    ❑ No ❑ No estoy seguro(a)

49. ¿Te has perforaste (excluyendo las orejas) o recibiste algún tatuaje en el cuerpo? ....... ❑ Sí    ❑ No ❑ Lo estoy pensando

## Emociones

50. ¿Te has divertido en las últimas dos semanas? ..................................... ❑ No ❑ Sí

51. Durante las últimas dos semanas, ¿te has sentido triste con frecuencia, o desganado, o como si no tuvieras nada que buscar en la mañana? ...................... ❑ Sí    ❑ No

52. ¿Alguna vez has seriamente pensado en el suicidio, hecho planes para hacerlo, o tratado de matarte? ........................................................................... ❑ Sí    ❑ No

53. ¿Alguna vez te han abusado físicamente, sexualmente, o emocionalmente? ............ ❑ Sí    ❑ No ❑ No estoy seguro(a)

54. ¿Haces cosas violentas cuando te enojas? ............................................. ❑ Sí    ❑ No

55. ¿Deseas tener una consulta profesional sobre algo que te está molestando? ............. ❑ Sí    ❑ No ❑ No estoy seguro(a)

## Circunstancias Especiales

56. En los últimos 12 meses, ¿estuviste con alguien que tiene tuberculosis? .................. ❑ Sí    ❑ No ❑ No estoy seguro(a)

57. ¿Te has quedado alguna noche en un refugio para desamparados, cárcel, o prisión juvenil? .......................................................................... ❑ Sí    ❑ No

58. ¿Has vivido en un hogar adoptivo o una casa para grupos de jóvenes? ................... ❑ Sí    ❑ No

## Sobre Tu Persona

59. ¿Cuáles son las cuatro palabras que mejor describen cómo eres? _____

60. Si pudieras cambiar algo en tu vida, o en tu persona, ¿qué cosa cambiarías?_____
_____

61. ¿De qué cosas quieres hablar hoy? _____

97-896:1.2M:11/97

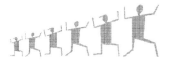

Date _____

Adolescent's name _____ Adolescent's birthday _____ Age _____

Parent/Guardian name _____ Relationship to adolescent _____

Your phone number: Home _____ Work _____

## Adolescent Health History

1. Is your adolescent allergic to any medicines?
   ☐ Yes  ☐ No   If yes, what medicines? _____

2. Please provide the following information about medicines your adolescent is taking.

| Name of medicine | Reason taken | How long taken |
|---|---|---|
| _____ | _____ | _____ |
| _____ | _____ | _____ |
| _____ | _____ | _____ |

3. Has your adolescent ever been hospitalized overnight?
   ☐ Yes  ☐ No   If yes, give the age at time of hospitalization and describe the problem.

   | Age | Problem |
   |---|---|
   | _____ | _____ |
   | _____ | _____ |

4. Has your adolescent ever had any serious injuries?
   ☐ Yes  ☐ No   If yes, please explain. _____

5. Have there been any changes in your adolescent's health during the past 12 months?
   ☐ Yes  ☐ No   If yes, please explain. _____

6. Please check (✔) whether your adolescent ever had any of the following health problems:
   If yes, at what age did the problem start:

| | Yes | No | Age | | Yes | No | Age |
|---|---|---|---|---|---|---|---|
| ADHD/learning disability | ☐ | ☐ | _____ | Headaches/migraines | ☐ | ☐ | _____ |
| Allergies/hayfever | ☐ | ☐ | _____ | Low iron in blood (anemia) | ☐ | ☐ | _____ |
| Asthma | ☐ | ☐ | _____ | Pneumonia | ☐ | ☐ | _____ |
| Bladder or kidney infections | ☐ | ☐ | _____ | Rheumatic fever or heart disease | ☐ | ☐ | _____ |
| Blood disorders/sickle cell anemia | ☐ | ☐ | _____ | Scoliosis (curved spine) | ☐ | ☐ | _____ |
| Cancer | ☐ | ☐ | _____ | Seizures/epilepsy | ☐ | ☐ | _____ |
| Chicken pox | ☐ | ☐ | _____ | Severe acne | ☐ | ☐ | _____ |
| Depression | ☐ | ☐ | _____ | Stomach problems | ☐ | ☐ | _____ |
| Diabetes | ☐ | ☐ | _____ | Tuberculosis (TB)/lung disease | ☐ | ☐ | _____ |
| Eating disorder | ☐ | ☐ | _____ | Mononucleosis (mono) | ☐ | ☐ | _____ |
| Emotional disorder | ☐ | ☐ | _____ | Other: _____ | ☐ | ☐ | _____ |
| Hepatitis (liver disease) | ☐ | ☐ | _____ | | | | |

7. Does this office or clinic have an up-to-date record of your adolescent's immunizations (record of "shots")?
   ☐ Yes  ☐ No  ☐ Not sure

## Family History

8. Some health problems are passed from one generation to the next. Have you or any of your adolescent's *blood* relatives (parents, grandparents, aunts, uncles, brothers or sisters), living or deceased, had any of the following problems? If the answer is "Yes," please state the age of the person when the problem occurred and his or her relationship to your adolescent.

| | Yes | No | Unsure | Age at Onset | Relationship |
|---|---|---|---|---|---|
| Allergies/asthma | ☐ | ☐ | ☐ | _____ | _____ |
| Arthritis | ☐ | ☐ | ☐ | _____ | _____ |
| Birth defects | ☐ | ☐ | ☐ | _____ | _____ |
| Blood disorders/sickle cell anemia | ☐ | ☐ | ☐ | _____ | _____ |

| | Yes | No | Unsure | Age at Onset | Relationship |
|---|---|---|---|---|---|
| Cancer (type_____) | ☐ | ☐ | ☐ | _____ | _____ |
| Depression | ☐ | ☐ | ☐ | _____ | _____ |
| Diabetes | ☐ | ☐ | ☐ | _____ | _____ |
| Drinking problem/alcoholism | ☐ | ☐ | ☐ | _____ | _____ |
| Drug addiction | ☐ | ☐ | ☐ | _____ | _____ |
| Endocrine/gland disease | ☐ | ☐ | ☐ | _____ | _____ |
| Heart attack or stroke *before* age 55 | ☐ | ☐ | ☐ | _____ | _____ |
| Heart attack or stroke *after* age 55 | ☐ | ☐ | ☐ | _____ | _____ |
| High blood pressure | ☐ | ☐ | ☐ | _____ | _____ |
| High cholesterol | ☐ | ☐ | ☐ | _____ | _____ |
| Kidney disease | ☐ | ☐ | ☐ | _____ | _____ |
| Learning disability | ☐ | ☐ | ☐ | _____ | _____ |
| Liver disease | ☐ | ☐ | ☐ | _____ | _____ |
| Mental health | ☐ | ☐ | ☐ | _____ | _____ |
| Mental retardation | ☐ | ☐ | ☐ | _____ | _____ |
| Migraine headaches | ☐ | ☐ | ☐ | _____ | _____ |
| Obesity | ☐ | ☐ | ☐ | _____ | _____ |
| Seiures/epilepsy | ☐ | ☐ | ☐ | _____ | _____ |
| Smoking | ☐ | ☐ | ☐ | _____ | _____ |
| Tuberculosis/lung disease | ☐ | ☐ | ☐ | _____ | _____ |

9. With whom does the adolescent live most of the time? *(Check all that apply.)*

☐ Both parents in same household   ☐ Stepmother   ☐ Sister(s)/ages _____
☐ Mother   ☐ Stepfather   ☐ Other _____
☐ Father   ☐ Guardian   ☐ Alone
☐ Other adult relative   ☐ Brother(s)/ages _____

10. In the past year, have there been any changes in your family? *(Check all that apply.)*
☐ Marriage   ☐ Loss of job   ☐ Births   ☐ Other _____
☐ Separation   ☐ Move to a new neighborhood   ☐ Serious illness
☐ Divorce   ☐ A new school or college   ☐ Deaths

**Parental/Guardian Concerns**

11. Please review the topics listed below. Check(✔) if you have a concern about your adolescent.

| | Concern About My Adolescent | | Concern About My Adolescent |
|---|---|---|---|
| Physical problems | ☐ | Guns/weapons | ☐ |
| Physical development | ☐ | School grades/absences/dropout | ☐ |
| Weight | ☐ | Smoking cigarettes/chewing tobacco | ☐ |
| Change of appetite | ☐ | Drug use | ☐ |
| Sleep patterns | ☐ | Alcohol use | ☐ |
| Diet/nutrition | ☐ | Dating/parties | ☐ |
| Amount of physical activity | ☐ | Sexual behavior | ☐ |
| Emotional development | ☐ | Unprotected sex | ☐ |
| Relationships with parents and family | ☐ | HIV/AIDS | ☐ |
| Choice of friends | ☐ | Sexual transmitted diseases (STDs) | ☐ |
| Self image or self worth | ☐ | Pregnancy | ☐ |
| Excessive moodiness or rebellion | ☐ | Sexual identity | |
| Depression | ☐ | (heterosexual/homosexual/bisexual) | ☐ |
| Lying, stealing, or vandalism | ☐ | Work or job | ☐ |
| Violence/gangs | ☐ | Other: _____ | ☐ |

12. What seems to be the greatest challenge for your teen? _____

13. What is it about your teen that makes you proud of him or her? _____

14. Is there something on your mind that you would like to talk about today?

   What is it? _____

15. Can we share your answers to Question 13 with your teen?   ☐ Yes   ☐ No

AA59:97-894:11/97

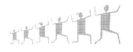

## Guía De Servicios Preventivos Para Los Adolescentes
## Cuestionario Para Padres o Guardianes

**Confidencial** (No le diremos a nadie lo que nos diga)

Fecha _____

Nombre del adolescente _____ Fecha de nacimiento _____ Edad _____

Nombre del Padre o Guardián _____ Su relación con el adolescente _____

Su número de teléfono: de casa ( _____ ) _____ del trabajo ( _____ ) _____

### Historial Médico del Adolescente

1. ¿Es su adolescente alérgico a alguna medicina?
   ☐ Sí ☐ No          Si la respuesta es *Sí*, ¿a cuál medicina? _____

2. Por favor, díganos qué medicinas está tomando su adolescente.

   | Nombre de la medicina | Razón para tomarla | Cuánto tiempo tiene tomándola |
   | --- | --- | --- |
   | _____ | _____ | _____ |
   | _____ | _____ | _____ |

3. ¿Alguna vez ha estado hospitalizado su adolescente?
   ☐ Sí ☐ No    Si la respuesta es *Sí*, escriba la edad que tenía y explique cuál era el problema.
   Edad         Problema
   _____  _____
   _____  _____

4. ¿Su adolescente alguna vez se ha lastimado seriamente?
   ☐ Sí ☐ No    Si su respuesta es *Sí*, por favor explique. _____

5. ¿Ha notado cambios en la salud de su adolescente en los últimos 12 meses?
   ☐ Sí ☐ No    Si su respuesta es *Sí*, por favor explique. _____

6. Por favor, marque (✓) si su adolescente alguna vez padeció de alguno de los siguientes problemas de salud. Si su respuesta es *Sí*, marque cuántos años tenía cuando comenzó el problema.

   | | Sí | No | Edad | | Sí | No | Edad |
   | --- | --- | --- | --- | --- | --- | --- | --- |
   | Problemas de aprendizaje/ADHD | ☐ | ☐ | ____ | Dolores de Cabeza/Migrañas | ☐ | ☐ | ____ |
   | Alergias | ☐ | ☐ | ____ | Falta de Hierro en la Sangre (anemia) | ☐ | ☐ | ____ |
   | Asma | ☐ | ☐ | ____ | Pulmonía | ☐ | ☐ | ____ |
   | Infección de la vejiga o de los riñones | ☐ | ☐ | ____ | Fiebre reumática o enfermed del corazón | ☐ | ☐ | ____ |
   | Enfermedad de la Sangre | ☐ | ☐ | ____ | Escoliosis (columna vertebral curva) | ☐ | ☐ | ____ |
   | Cáncer | ☐ | ☐ | ____ | Convulsiones/Epilepsia | ☐ | ☐ | ____ |
   | Varicela | ☐ | ☐ | ____ | Acné | ☐ | ☐ | ____ |
   | Depresión | ☐ | ☐ | ____ | Problemas Estomacales | ☐ | ☐ | ____ |
   | Diabetes | ☐ | ☐ | ____ | Tuberculosis/enfermedad del pulmón | ☐ | ☐ | ____ |
   | Problemas Alimenticios | ☐ | ☐ | ____ | Mononucleosis | ☐ | ☐ | ____ |
   | Problemas Emocionales | ☐ | ☐ | ____ | Otra(s): _____ | ☐ | ☐ | ____ |
   | Hepatitis (enfermedad del hígado) | ☐ | ☐ | ____ | | | | |

7. ¿Tiene esta clínica toda la información sobre las vacunas de su adolescente?
   ☐ Sí ☐ No ☐ No estoy seguro

### Historial Familiar

8. Algunos problemas de salud se pasan de generación a generación. ¿Hay alún pariente biológico, de su adolescente (padres, abuelos, tíos, o hermanos), que haya tenido alguna de las siguientes enfermedades? Incluya parientes vivos y difuntos. Si la respuesta es *Sí*, marque cuántos años tenía la persona cuando empezó el problema y su relación con su adolescente.

   | | Sí | No | No estoy seguro | Edad cuando empezó | Relación con el adolescente |
   | --- | --- | --- | --- | --- | --- |
   | Alergias/Asma | ☐ | ☐ | ☐ | _____ | _____ |
   | Artritis | ☐ | ☐ | ☐ | _____ | _____ |
   | Defectos de Nacimiento | ☐ | ☐ | ☐ | _____ | _____ |
   | Enfermedad de sangre | ☐ | ☐ | ☐ | _____ | _____ |
   | Cáncer (de qué tipo_____ ) | ☐ | ☐ | ☐ | _____ | _____ |

Voltee la página

## Confidencial

Nombre _____

| | Sí | No | No estoy seguro | Edad cuando empezó | Relación con el adolescente |
|---|---|---|---|---|---|
| Depresión | ❑ | ❑ | ❑ | _____ | _____ |
| Diabetes | ❑ | ❑ | ❑ | _____ | _____ |
| Problema con la bebida/Alcoholismo | ❑ | ❑ | ❑ | _____ | _____ |
| Adicción a drogas | ❑ | ❑ | ❑ | _____ | _____ |
| Enfermedad del sistema endocrino | ❑ | ❑ | ❑ | _____ | _____ |
| Ataques al Corazón o Embolias antes de los 55 años | ❑ | ❑ | ❑ | _____ | _____ |
| Ataques al Corazón o Embolias después de los 55 años | ❑ | ❑ | ❑ | _____ | _____ |
| Presión Alta | ❑ | ❑ | ❑ | _____ | _____ |
| Alto Nivel de Colesterol | ❑ | ❑ | ❑ | _____ | _____ |
| Enfermedad de los Riñones | ❑ | ❑ | ❑ | _____ | _____ |
| Problemas de Aprendizaje | ❑ | ❑ | ❑ | _____ | _____ |
| Enfermedad del Hígado | ❑ | ❑ | ❑ | _____ | _____ |
| Salud Mental | ❑ | ❑ | ❑ | _____ | _____ |
| Retardo Mental | ❑ | ❑ | ❑ | _____ | _____ |
| Migrañas | ❑ | ❑ | ❑ | _____ | _____ |
| Obesidad | ❑ | ❑ | ❑ | _____ | _____ |
| Convulsiones/Epilepsia | ❑ | ❑ | ❑ | _____ | _____ |
| Fumar | ❑ | ❑ | ❑ | _____ | _____ |
| Tuberculosis/enfermedad del pulmón | ❑ | ❑ | ❑ | _____ | _____ |

9. ¿Con quién vive el adolescente la mayor parte del año? (Marque todas las que sean ciertas)
- ❑ Ambos padres en la misma casa
- ❑ Madre
- ❑ Padre
- ❑ Otro pariente adulto
- ❑ Madrastra
- ❑ Padrastro
- ❑ Guardián Legal
- ❑ Hermanos/edades _____
- ❑ Hermanas/edades _____
- ❑ Otra persona _____
- ❑ Solo

10. En estos últimos 12 meses, ¿han habido cambios importantes en su familia? (Marque todos los que sean ciertos.)
- ❑ Matrimonios
- ❑ Separaciones
- ❑ Divorcios
- ❑ Alguien perdió el trabajo
- ❑ Mudanzas a otros vecindarios
- ❑ Cambio de escuela o universidad
- ❑ Nacimientos
- ❑ Enfermedades graves
- ❑ Muertes
- ❑ Otros_____

## Preocupaciones de los padres o guardián

11. Por favor, fíjese en los temas que le damos a continuación. Marque (✓) si tiene usted alguna preocupación sobre algún tema con respecto a su adolescente.

| | Me preocupa | | Me preocupa |
|---|---|---|---|
| Problemas físicos | ❑ | Pistolas/armas | ❑ |
| Desarrollo físico | ❑ | Malas notas escolares/ausencias/abandono de estudios | ❑ |
| Peso | ❑ | Fumar cigarrillos/mascar tabaco | ❑ |
| Cambios en su apetito | ❑ | Uso de drogas | ❑ |
| Hábitos de dormir | ❑ | Uso de bebidas alcohólicas | ❑ |
| Hábitos de comer/nutrición | ❑ | Noviazgos/Fiestas | ❑ |
| La cantidad de actividad física | ❑ | Conducta sexual | ❑ |
| Desarrollo emocional | ❑ | Relaciones sexuales sin protección | ❑ |
| Su relación con sus padres y familia | ❑ | VIH-SIDA | ❑ |
| Tipo de amigos que tiene | ❑ | Enfermedades Transmitidas Sexualmente | ❑ |
| Auto-proyección o auto-estima | ❑ | El embarazo | ❑ |
| Cambios exagerados de carácter o rebelión | ❑ | Identidad Sexual (heterosexual, homosexual, bisexual) | ❑ |
| Depresión | ❑ | El trabajo u ocupación | ❑ |
| Mentir, robar, o vandalismo | ❑ | Otra_____ | |
| Violencia/pandillas | ❑ | | |

12. ¿Cuáles son los retos personales más difíciles para su adolescente? _____

13. ¿Qué lo enorgullece de su adolescente? _____

14. Hoy, ¿Quisiera hablarnos sobre algo en especial? ¿Que? _____

15. ¿Nos permite mostrarle a su adolescente su respuesta a la Pregunta #13?  ❑ Sí   ❑ No

# Performing a Mental Status Exam

If a child is suspected to have a mental health problem after screening and clinical interview, it is important to perform a mental status exam along with a thorough physical exam to rule out potential physical causes of mental health problems. For example, children or teens with depression could have underlying iron deficiency or hypothyroidism. Components of the mental status exam include the following:

- Appearance (e.g., how is the child dressed and groomed?)
- Attitude and interaction (e.g., is the child cooperative, guarded, or avoidant?)
- Activity level/behavior (e.g., is the child calm, active, or restless; are psychomotor activity, abnormal movements, and tics present?)
- Speech (e.g., is the child's speech loud or quiet, flat in tone or full of intonation, slow or rushed? How are words formed? Does the child understand what is being said to him or her? Does the child express himself or herself appropriately?)
- Thought processes (e.g., coherent, disorganized, flight of ideas [rapid skipping from topic to topic], blocking [inability to fill memory gaps], loosening associations [the shifting of topics quickly even though unrelated; echolalia [mocking repetition of another person's words]; perseveration: [repetition of verbal or motor response])
- Thought content (including delusions [false, irrational beliefs, such as "I am superman"]; obsessions [persistent thoughts or impulses];  perceptual disorders [including hallucinations (altered sensory perceptions, such as hearing voices inside or outside his/her head that others are unaware); phobias [irrational fears]; hypochondriasis [excessive worry about personal health without an actual reason]
- Impulse control (e.g., is the child able to control aggressive, hostile, and sexual impulses)
- Mood/affect (e.g., depressed, anxious, flat, ambivalent, fearful, irritable, elated, euphoric, inappropriate)
- Suicidal and/or homicidal behavior/ideation
- Cognitive functioning (e.g., orientation to surroundings, attention span/concentration, memory [recent and remote]; ability to abstract; insight/judgment)
- Parent-child interaction (e.g., warm, nurturing, confliction, rejecting, appropriate use of limit setting, in tune with child's feeling/needs, affectionate, eye contact, and other body language)

# Example of a Mental Status Assessment Write-up

Shannon is a well-groomed, healthy-appearing, overweight adolescent who is cooperative and pleasant in her conversation. She sits calmly without making abnormal movements and makes good eye contact. Her rate and quality of speech are normal. Her thought processes are generally well organized and free of delusions. Shannon states that she can go quickly from a 0 to 10 in terms of anger. It is evident that she has a pattern of depressive cognitive thinking as she degrades herself frequently.

On a scale of 0 to 10, Shannon rates her depression as 4-5 on average and talks about the fact that she sometimes worries, especially about how other people view her. She denies hallucinations or any sleep problems. Shannon states that she needs help with anger management. She has poor impulse control as evidenced by frequent anger outbursts in her home. Shannon denies suicidal or homicidal ideations. She has some insight into her problems and talks about her desire to be a landscape designer. Short- and long-term memories are intact.

# The Big Secret about Well-Child Visits for Parents

## Understanding the Well-Child Visit

Every day, "healthy" children are brought to doctors and nurse practitioners for well-child visits. Leading pediatric authorities recommend 22 routine visits, ideally beginning with a prenatal visit and continuing throughout infancy, childhood, and adolescence. The purpose of these visits is to help families keep children healthy as well as to pick up early signs of potential problems. These visits are recognized as being so important to a child's health that both private and public insurance companies pay for them. This is because childhood is a unique period of time to lay the foundation for a person's health throughout life.

Yet a funny thing sometimes happens during these visits. The most important part of the visit gets overlooked. Many parents don't even realize that both they and their healthcare provider are forgetting to talk about the biggest threats to their child's well-being.

Many things happen during these visits. Many of the activities are very visible, like weighing a child and providing him or her with necessary immunizations. But sometimes, the most important part of the visit, the part that is not so easy to see, gets forgotten. That is the part of the visit that should be spent talking to your doctor or nurse practitioner about how your child is growing emotionally and mentally and the important role that behavior plays in keeping your child healthy.

Unlike 100 years ago, the greatest threats faced by children in this country today are not infection and physical illnesses. The Surgeon General and others have often called attention to the real risks to children's health today. **Children's health today is threatened most by behavior** – their own behaviors, the behaviors of their families and friends, or sometimes the behavior of strangers. Many children and adolescents die from accidents and injuries, from homicide, and suicide. One in 4 has a mental health disorder and many more have behavior problems that interfere with their family relationships, their friendships, and their performance in school. Mental health problems appear in families of all social classes and backgrounds. Child mental health problems often continue into adulthood and worsen if untreated. Yet, more is known today than ever before about how to recognize early mental health problems in children and how to help them during the critical childhood years. It is most important that you talk to your healthcare provider about your child's behavior on a regular basis and share your concerns.

There is nothing to be ashamed of if your child has an emotional or behavior problem. The sooner you share your concerns with your child's doctor or nurse practitioner, the faster your child can be helped.

**Please see next page to view a list of steps you can take to keep your child healthy.**

# Parents: Did you remember to talk to your doctor/nurse practitioner today about your child's behavior and emotions?

*Remember:*

*Both parents and healthcare providers have a role to play in keeping children mentally and physically healthy.*

## How Can Parents Assure This Happens

1. Expect your pediatric healthcare provider to talk to you routinely about your child's behavior and emotions. Many doctors and nurse practitioners will use behavioral screening tools at every visit to help recognize when children are having more difficulties than usual.

2. Call or make an appointment to talk to your healthcare provider when you have concerns about your child's behavior or emotions.

3. Some concerns can be dealt with in a single visit, but most will require follow-up calls or appointments. Following up is most important.

4. Some pediatric healthcare providers have more experience in behavior/mental health management than others. After taking a careful history, some providers may suggest that you be referred to a mental health clinician. But others will talk to you about some short-term interventions they may be able to provide, such as:

   a. Formal screening for mental health problems and strengths
   b. Discussions to help you and your child better understand the problem
   c. Brief solution-focused counseling sessions that help you and your child manage the problem
   d. Participation in group sessions with other parents or children

5. If the problem is not getting better or seems to be getting worse, do not hesitate to ask your healthcare provider for a referral to someone with expertise in the mental healthcare of children.

6. Keep your pediatric provider informed about your child's progress even after referral to a specialist. Your pediatric primary care provider has an important role to play in helping you to advocate for your child's continued mental and physical health.

# Internet Resources

## American Academy of Child and Adolescent Psychiatry
www.aacap.org
This Web site provides excellent information on the assessment and treatment of child and adolescent mental health disorders. Handouts addressing a multitude of problems (i.e., *Facts for Families*) are available.

## KidsHealth
www.kidshealth.org
This is an outstanding Web site that contains health information for healthcare providers, parents, teens, and children. Many of the topics relate to emotions and behaviors (e.g., anxiety, fears, depression) and are developmentally sensitive to specific age groups. Physicians and other healthcare providers review all material before it is posted on this Web site.

## National Association of Pediatric Nurse Practitioners' (NAPNAP) KySS Program
www.napnap.org
This site can be accessed to keep abreast of all ongoing and new initiatives of the KySS program. Some handouts for downloading and use in practice are available to assist families in dealing with stressful situations (e.g., war, terrorism). Proceedings of the First National KySS Institute on Mental Health Screening, Intervention, and Health Promotion for Pediatric and Adolescent Primary Care and School Health Providers are available on CD-ROM for purchase. Email info@napnap.org or call NAPNAP at 856-857-9700.

## Pediatric Development and Behavior
http://www.dbpeds.org/
This outstanding Web site is targeted to professionals who are interested in child development and behavior, especially in medical settings. It is an outstanding site that houses a variety of screening tools as well as educational handouts on developmental and behavioral problems that are downloadable for use in practice. There is a learning section that features "the toolbox," which is a link to special articles, features, keywords, and evidence. There is also a practice section that emphasizes practical information and tools to support primary care and specialty practice.

# References

American Medical Association (1994). Guidelines for adolescent preventive services.
Available at http://www.ama-ssn.org/ama/pub/category/2280.html.

Jellinek, M., Patel, B.P., & Froehle, M. (2002). *Bright Futures in Practice: Mental Health- Vol I. Practice Guide*. Arlington, VA: National Center for Education in Maternal and Child Health.

Jellinek, M. & Patel, B.P., & Froehle, M. (2002). *Bright Futures in Practice: Mental Health- Vol II. Tool Kit*. Arlington, VA: National Center for Education in Maternal and Child Health.

Kaye, D.L., Montgomery, M.E., & Munson, S. (2002). Child and adolescent mental health. Philadelphia, PA: Lippincott.

Melnyk, B.M., Brown, H., Jones, D.C., Kreipe, R., & Novak, J. (2003). Improving the mental/psychosocial health of U.S. children and adolescents. Outcomes and implementation strategies from the national KySS summit. *Journal of Pediatric Healthcare*, 17 (6: Supplement 1): S1- S24.

Moldenhauer, Z. & Melnyk, B.M. (in press for 2006). Assessment and management of common mental health disorders in children and adolescents. In N. Ryan-Wenger (Ed), NAPNAP/AFPNP: Core Curriculum for Pediatric Nurse Practitioners. Philadelphia, PA: Elsevier.

**Section 2**
Diagnosing, Managing, and Preventing Mental Health Disorders
**Bernadette Melnyk**

Section 2
Diagnosing, Managing,
and Preventing

# Diagnosing Mental Health Disorders

Mental health disorders are diagnosed according to the classification system published in the *Diagnostic and Statistical Manual of Mental Disorders (Fourth Edition)* (DSM-IV) by the American Psychiatric Association, which includes the following categories:

- Axis 1: Psychological disorders (e.g., major depressive disorder, generalized anxiety disorder)
- Axis 2: Psychological disorders (e.g., borderline personality)/mental retardation
- Axis 3: General medical conditions (e.g., asthma, diabetes)
- Axis 4: Psychosocial and environmental problems (e.g., problems with primary support group, social environment; educational problems; occupational problems; housing problems; economic problems; problems with access to healthcare services, problems related to interaction with the legal system)
- Axis 5: Global assessment of functioning (GAF) (e.g., psychological, social, and work functioning); a score is given on a scale of 100 (superior functioning) to 0 (inadequate information). For example, a score of 21-50 would indicate symptoms of serious impairment in social, occupational, or school functioning

It is important to exercise much caution when placing DSM-IV diagnoses on children and adolescents, as stigma and labeling can place additional burdens upon an already stressed family system, especially if the diagnosis is not accurate. However, correctly identifying a diagnosis and beginning early intervention as well as providing comprehensive psycho-education can be of enormous relief and assist the child and family in obtaining positive outcomes. Before a diagnosis is made, it is necessary to gain collateral information from multiple sources (e.g., the child's parents and school teachers) and to conduct a comprehensive interview with the child and family. If the diagnosis is in doubt and/or the disorder is complex or not responsive to early intervention strategies, it is critical to have the child seen and concurrently managed by a mental health provider (e.g., psychiatrist, psychiatric mental health nurse practitioner, or psychologist).

# General Approach to the Management of Mental Health Disorders in Children and Adolescents

Based upon the assessment, a decision must be made to:

- Intervene
- Consult with a mental health professional
- Refer to a mental health professional (it is important to know the mental health specialists in your area and preferably to send the family to someone in close proximity; follow-up is critical to assure that the family has adhered to the referral)

  Possible referrals include:
  - Outpatient services
  - Partial hospital services
  - Inpatient services
  - Emergency and urgent care services
  - Youth emergency services, lifeline, preventive services of the department of social services

In making a decision about management, consider severity, persistence, and resistance to change.

Once a mental health problem is identified, support of and therapeutic communications with the family are critical.

Treating a child/teen for a mental health problem typically requires more than 1 person or system.

Many early interventions, especially with young children, are parent-focused.

School-age and teen interventions need to be skill oriented, and it is best to teach the skills to both children and parents.

## Psycho-education

Counseling parents and children/teens about what to expect in dealing with a particular condition is critical, as it will assist them in coping with the condition and adhering to treatment.

## Psychosocial Interventions

More evidence exists for psychosocial interventions (e.g., cognitive behavior skills therapy) than for any other type of intervention in support of their efficacy for treating mood, anxiety, and behavior disorders.

Lewinsohn and Clark's "Adolescent Coping with Stress and Coping with Depression" programs are evidence-based and downloadable for use without permission or cost at www.kpchr.org/public/acwd/acwd.html.

## Psychopharmacology

Medications supported as the most effective, on the basis of clinical trials with children and teens, include stimulant medications for attention-deficit/hyperactivity disorder (ADHD) and selective serotonin reuptake inhibitors (SSRIs) for obsessive-compulsive disorder and moderate to severe major depressive disorder. However, **medication alone is usually not fully effective in treating a mental health disorder**. A combination of medication with therapy/counseling typically leads to the best outcomes. Risperidone also has been empirically supported as an effective treatment for autism.

General rule of thumb when starting medication in children and teens: **Start Low, Go Slow!**

Providers without in-depth psychopharmacology education and skills training should be extremely cautious about prescribing medications for mental health disorders in children and teens without consultation from a child psychiatrist or psychiatric nurse practitioner.

Evidence-based management guidelines for some mental health disorders in children and adolescents can be found at www.guideline.gov; this is the National Guideline Clearinghouse for evidence-based clinical practice guidelines, sponsored by the Agency for Health Care Research and Quality and the American Medical Association. For information about how to critically appraise evidence-based guidelines, see Melnyk and Fineout-Overholt (2005).

# Prevention of Mental Health/
# Psychosocial Morbidities in Children and Teens

Prevention of mental health disorders should occur at the primary, secondary, and tertiary levels. Interventions should target the family, school, and community.

Primary prevention must start during pregnancy or at birth with parenting education and support (e.g., anticipatory guidance about normal developmental milestones and characteristics, temperament, discipline, and positive parenting strategies to facilitate self-esteem and close relationships). Remember that it is much easier to prevent behaviors that have never started than to curtail negative patterns. It is never too early to begin parent effectiveness training.

## *Parent Effectiveness Training as a Preventive and Early Intervention Strategy*

Important tips to provide to parents:

- Provide positive reinforcement/praise: "Catch children being good!"
- Provide specific praise (e.g., "I like the way you brushed your teeth without me telling you to today" instead of "You are a good girl").
- Promote independence and age-appropriate control.
- Set age-appropriate limits.
- Reward cooperative behavior (e.g., special time together, stickers).
- Provide age-appropriate independence and competencies.
- Give gradual increases in work responsibilities with increasing age.
- Allow children to make choices.
- Allow children to struggle some with challenges to build their coping strategies.
- Do not rush to answer questions for children.
- Help children learn to problem-solve and find resources to address their challenges.
- Define position on at-risk behaviors (e.g., zero tolerance for drug or alcohol use).
- Avoid double standards (e.g., "Do as I say, not as I do"), as modeling is a powerful learning mechanism.
- Don't make excuses for children/teens. (If parents think there is a problem, there usually is.)
- Frequently communicate expectations to children regarding behaviors and school performance.
- Become acquainted with their children's friends and the parents of their children's friends (hold meetings to determine group rules).
- Provide parents with excellent resources for parenting (see section Web sites and other resources).
- Caution parents to prevent their children/teens from watching R-rated movies, especially children under 13 years of age.
- Help parents to assist their children in dealing with the current stressful events in their lives and in our society.
- Encourage parents to take time for themselves to rest or relax, and to seek counseling if highly stressed, anxious, or depressed; emphasize to them that their mood state will affect their children.

- Emphasize the importance of daily physical activity and exercise in releasing stress and anxiety for all family members.
- Encourage family activities and outings.

## Important Information about Limit-Setting for Parents

- All feelings are okay; all behaviors are not.
- Work on only 1 or 2 limits at a time.
- Make sure that consequences are age appropriate.
- Follow through on limits set.

## Teach Parents How to Help Their School-Age Children and Teens

- Problem-solve
    - Identify the problem.
    - Identify the cause of the problem.
    - Generate solutions.
    - Discuss the consequence of each solution.
    - Choose a solution and put it into action.

- Teach parents structured choices
    - Give children at least 2 choices about something that needs to happen. This increases decision-making ability, cooperation, independence, and self-esteem. For example: "Do you want to do your homework before or after dinner today? You decide -- it's up to you."

- Develop positive patterns of thinking
    - Teach the thinking, behaving, and emotion triangle (i.e., how you think affects how you behave and how you feel. If you think you are stupid, you will feel depressed and not attempt to do better in school). It is necessary to stop the negative thought and turn it into a positive one (e.g., "Okay, I may not have done as well on my math test as I should have, but I'm good at English." The consequence is feeling emotionally better).

- Control anger
    - Help the child identify anger triggers and cues as well as implement cool-down strategies, such as:
        - Counting to 10 or saying the alphabet
        - Diaphragmatic breathing
        - Walking away
        - Positive self-talk (e.g., "I am calming down")
        - Writing it down
        - Talking it out
        - Listening to music
        - Communicating his/her anger to the person in appropriate ways
        - Telling the other person he or she is angry, using "I" instead of "You" statements

- Channeling the anger in appropriate ways (e.g., use physical activity)
- Learning to accept no for an answer or unchangeable situations (e.g., you cannot change other people, only how to respond to them)

## Parents and Children/Teens Need to Know How to Access Resources

- Children/teens and parents need to learn where to turn for help and information.
- It is critical to know your community resources.
- Reinforce to children/teens and parents that you deal with their mental and emotional health just as you deal with their physical health.
- Encourage families to use multiple resources (e.g., the Internet, books, school staff, healthcare professionals, extended family, and mental health professionals).

## Other Preventive Strategies

- Screen for mental health/psychosocial morbidities at every healthcare encounter.
- Assess parenting competence, style, stressors, and presence of mental health problems.
- Raise awareness of these problems (e.g., use posters in practice settings, distribute handouts, teach parenting classes).
- Build developmental assets in children/teen and parents as well communities (e.g., teach effective communication strategies, problem-solving skills, refusal skills, and coping strategies; provide children and teens with opportunities for involvement in community education).
- Implement preventive strategies for children and teens at highest risk for psychopathology and for those who have experienced traumatic events, including motor vehicle accidents, hospitalization, and rape, as well as family and neighborhood violence.
- Encourage parents to be actively involved in their children's lives, and to monitor their activities (e.g., who, what, when, and where) as well as the things that they are reading, watching, and listening.
- Emphasize to parents the importance of mentoring and modeling healthy behaviors.
- Advise parents to require 48-hour advance notice for sleeping over at a friend's house, as most drug and alcohol parties come together at the last minute.
- Encourage parents to spend special time with their children/teens and to listen to them.
- Facilitate mentors for children/teens, as those who have mentors are less likely to use illegal drugs and alcohol and are less likely to skip school.
- Encourage service to others, such as belonging to sport/club/hobby/religious groups.
- Provide opportunities for children to be successful; encourage mastery of skill development; teach coping and problem-solving strategies as well as refusal skills; build relationships with youth.
- Teach children coping and problem-solving skills (e.g., encourage journaling and creating expression with school-age children and teens).
- Detect abuse and neglect early, address poverty, build strong families with supports/resources.
- Use quality resources to promote mental health in your state.

# Internet Resources

### Adventures in Parenting
www.healthfinder.gov/docs/doc06425.htm
This evidence-based publication for parents was developed by the National Institute of Child Health and Human Development. This booklet incorporates evidence from 30 years of research on effective parenting techniques to stimulate healthy development. It can be downloaded free of charge. You can also call the NICHD Information Resource Center at 800-370-2943.

### Bright Futures Handouts for Families
www.brightfutures.org/
Encounter forms for each well-child visit throughout childhood and adolescence can be accessed at this site.

### The Children's Mental Health Resource Kit: Promoting Children's Mental Health Screens and Assessments
www.cdfhealth@childrensdefense.org
This Resource Kit can be accessed on the Web site or by calling 202-662-3575.

### Creating Opportunities for Parent Empowerment (COPE)
http://copeforhope.com/
This Web site provides a series of evidence-based intervention materials that can be easily administered in clinical practice settings, aimed at parents with children experiencing marital separation or divorce, hospitalization, critical illness, and those experiencing the birth of a premature infant.

### A Guide to Positive Youth Development
http://www.human.cornell.edu/actforyouth
This is an excellent resource for parents and communities to guide them in assisting children to build developmental assets.

### Parent Soup
www.parentsoup.com/
This is an excellent Web site for parents that contain information about what to expect at each stage of development.

# References

Kaye, D.L., Montgomery, M.E., & Munson, S. (2002). Child and adolescent mental health. Philadelphia, Pa: Lippincott.

Jellinek, M., Patel, B.P., & Froehle, M. (2002). *Bright Futures in Practice: Mental Health- Vol I. Practice Guide*. Arlington, VA: National Center for Education in Maternal and Child Health.

Jellinek, M. Patel, B.P., & Froehle, M. (2002). *Bright Futures in Practice: Mental Health- Vol II. Tool Kit*. Arlington, VA: National Center for Education in Maternal and Child Health.

Melnyk, B.M., Brown, H., Jones, D.C., Kreipe, R., & Novak, J. (2003). Improving the mental/psychosocial health of U.S. children and adolescents. Outcomes and implementation strategies from the national KySS summit. *Journal of Pediatric Healthcare*, 17 (6 Supplement 1): S1- S24.

Melnyk, B.M. & Fineout-Overholt, E. (2005). *Evidence-Based Practice in Nursing & Healthcare. A Guide to Best Practice*. Philadelphia, Pa: Lippincott Williams & Wilkins.

Moldenhauer, Z. & Melnyk, B.M. (in press for 2006). Assessment and management of common mental health disorders in children and adolescents. In N. Ryan-Wenger (Ed), NAPNAP/AFPNP: Core Curriculum for Pediatric Nurse Practitioners. Philadelphia, PA: Elsevier

# Information for Healthcare Providers about Anxiety Disorders

## Quick Facts

- Fears and anxiety are a normal part of a child's development, but they should not interfere with functioning.
- Anxiety disorders are among the most common mental health problems in children and teens.
- Children and teens with anxiety disorders experience severe and persistent distress that interferes with their daily functioning; often these disorders are significantly under-reported and under-diagnosed.
- Parents describe these children as "worriers."
- Somatic complaints are very common (e.g., stomach pain, headaches, chest pain, and fatigue).
- Comorbidities are the rule and not the exception, such as depression, attention-deficit/hyperactivity disorder (ADHD), and substance abuse.
- Children with anxiety disorders are often misdiagnosed with ADHD.
- Somatic complaints, such as stomach pain, headaches, chest pain, and fatigue are common (See Table 3.1 for common signs of anxiety).

## Table 3.1 Common Signs of Anxiety in Children and Teens:

| Physical | Behavioral | Cognitive |
|---|---|---|
| Restlessness and irritability (very common in younger children) | Escape/avoidant behaviors | "What if...?" (cognitive distortions, negativistic thinking) |
| Headaches | Crying | Catastrophic thoughts (threat bias, low perceived control) |
| Stomachaches, nausea, vomiting, diarrhea | Clinging to/fear of separation from parents | |
| Fatigue | Soft voice | |
| Palpitations, increased heart rate, increased blood pressure | Variations in speech | |
| Hyperventilation or shortness of breath | Nail-biting | |
| Muscle tension | Thumb-sucking | |
| Difficulty sleeping | Vigilance and scanning | |
| Dizziness, tingling, weakness | Freezing | |
| Tremors | Regressions (bedwetting, temper tantrums) | |

## Anxiety Spectrum Diagnoses

- Separation anxiety disorder
- Generalized anxiety disorder (includes overanxious disorder of childhood)
- Specific phobia
- Social phobia
- Panic disorder
- Acute stress disorder
- Posttraumatic stress disorder
- Obsessive compulsive disorder

## Critical History-Taking Questions

- Is the anxiety appropriate for the age of the child or teen?
- Has this child/teen experienced a traumatic event (e.g., has the child been a witness to domestic violence, physical/sexual abuse)?
- Does the anxiety interfere with the child's daily functioning (e.g., recent school attendance and grades) and sleep?
- Is there a history of recent stressful life events, marital transition, or family members with mental health disorders?

## Medical Conditions to be Ruled Out

- Hypoglycemia
- Hyperthyroidism
- Pheochromocytoma
- Seizure disorder
- Cardiac arrhythmia
- Migraine headaches
- Brain tumor
- Hypoxia

## Medications/Drugs That May Cause Anxiety

- Caffeine
- Nicotine
- Antihistamine
- Antiasthmatics (e.g., theophylline)
- Marijuana
- Sympathomimetics (e.g., nasal decongestants such as pseudoephedrine)
- Stimulants (including cocaine)
- Steroids
- Antipsychotics (e.g., for treatment of akathisia)
- SSRIs (e.g., *Celexa, Prozac, Luvox, Paxil, Zoloft*)

## Treatment

- Careful assessment
- Educate parents and children about common signs and symptoms
- Behavioral intervention
- Individual therapy (cognitive behavioral therapy, interpersonal therapy, play therapy)
- Family therapy
- Environmental changes: promote optimal sleep habits, decrease stressors
- Pharmacological intervention
- First-line: antidepressants/anti-anxiety agents (SSRIs) and buspirone
- Second-line: venlafaxine and benzodiazepines
- Alternatives: alpha-adrenergic agents, beta blockers, or antihistamines
- Pharmacological intervention (See Table 3.2 for medications used to treat pediatric anxiety disorders)

## Table 3.2 Medication Guide for Pediatric Anxiety Disorders

| Medication | Indications | Side Effects | Dosing | | |
|---|---|---|---|---|---|
| | | | Initial (mg) | Range (mg/day) | Schedule |
| Selective Serotonin Reuptake Inhibitors (SSRIs) | First-line treatment<br><br>Nonaddictive<br><br>Well tolerated | Nausea<br>Diarrhea<br>Insomnia<br>Somnolence<br>Headaches<br>Activation<br>Sexual dysfunction<br>Sweating<br>Tremor | | Use the lowest dose | |
| Citalopram | | | 5-20 QD | 10-60 | QD |
| Fluoxetine | | | 5-20 QAM | 10-80 | QD |
| Fluvoxamine | | | 12.5-50 QHS | 50-300 | QD-BID |
| Paroxetine | | | 5-10 mg QD | 10-60 | QD-BID |
| Sertraline | | | 12.5-25 QAM | 50-200 | QD-BID |
| Buspirone | First-line treatment for generalized anxiety<br><br>Nonaddictive<br><br>Well tolerated | Headache<br>Nausea<br>Dizziness<br>Lightheadedness<br>Somnolence | 5BID | 5-60 | BID-TID |
| Benzodiazepines<br><br>Diazepam<br>Clonazepam<br>Lorazepam | Second-line treatment<br><br>Addiction potential and cognitive blunting<br><br>Time-limited circumstances | Sedation<br>Cognitive blunting<br>Dizziness<br>Ataxia<br>Memory disturbance<br>Constipation<br>Diplopia<br>Hypotension | 1-2 HS<br>0.125-0.5<br>0.125-0.5 BID | 0.25-4<br>0.125-3<br>0.125-4 | HS-BID<br>HS-BID<br>HS-BID |

*Adapted from: Kutcher, S. Practical Child and Adolescent Psychopharmacology (2002). Cambridge, Mass: Cambridge University Press.*

**Note:** Caution must be exercised when prescribing SSRIs to children and adolescents with psychiatric disorders, as studies have shown an increased risk for suicidal thinking and behavior (suicidality) in the first few months after starting treatment. Patients started on SSRIs should be observed closely for worsening of symptoms, suicidality, or unusual changes in behavior. Families should be advised to monitor for these signs/symptoms and alert their provider if present.

# DSM-IV Criteria for Generalized Anxiety Disorder

The following is a list of the DSM-IV criteria for generalized anxiety disorder:

A.  Excessive anxiety and worry (apprehensive expectation), occurring more days than not for at least 6 months, about a number of events or activities (such as work or school performance).

B.  The person finds it difficult to control the worry.

C.  The anxiety and worry are associated with 3 (or more) of the following 6 symptoms (with at least some symptoms present for more days than not for the past 6 months).  Note: Only 1 item is required in children.

> Restlessness or feeling keyed up or on edge
>
> Being easily fatigued
>
> Difficulty concentrating or mind going blank
>
> Irritability
>
> Muscle tension
>
> Sleep disturbance (difficulty falling or staying asleep, or restless, unsatisfying sleep)

D.  The focus of the anxiety and worry is not confined to features of an Axis I disorder, e.g., the anxiety or worry is not about having a panic attack (as in a panic disorder), being embarrassed in public (as in social phobia), being contaminated (as in obsessive-compulsive disorder), being away from home or close relatives (as in separation anxiety disorder), gaining weight (as in anorexia nervosa), having multiple physical complaints (as in somatization disorder), or having a serious illness (as in hypochondriasis), and the anxiety and worry do not occur exclusively during posttraumatic stress disorder.

E.  The anxiety, worry, or physical symptoms cause clinically significant distress or impairment in social, occupational, or other important areas of functioning.

F.  The disturbance is not due to the direct physiological effects of a substance (e.g., a drug of abuse, a medication) or a general medical condition (e.g., hyperthyroidism) and does not occur exclusively during a mood disorder, a psychotic disorder, or a pervasive developmental disorder.

## DIAGNOSTIC FEATURES

The essential feature of generalized anxiety disorder is excessive anxiety and worry (apprehensive expectation), occurring more days than not for a period of at least 6 months, about a number of events or activities (criterion A).  The individual finds it difficult to control the worry (criterion B).  The anxiety and worry are accompanied by at least 3 additional symptoms from a list that includes restlessness, being easily fatigued, difficulty concentrating, irritability, muscle tension, and disturbed sleep (only 1 additional symptom is required in children) (criterion C).

The focus of the anxiety and worry is not confined to features of another Axis I disorder such as having a panic attack (as in panic disorder), being embarrassed in public (as in social phobia), being contaminated (as in obsessive-compulsive disorder), being away from home or close relatives (as in separation anxiety disorder), gaining weight (as in anorexia nervosa), having multiple physical complaints (as in somatization disorder), or having a serious illness (as in hypochondriasis), and the anxiety and worry do not occur exclusively during posttraumatic stress disorder (criterion D).

Although individuals with generalized anxiety disorder may not always identify the worries as "excessive," they report subjective distress due to constant worry, have difficulty controlling the worry, or experience-related impairment in social, occupational, or other important areas of functioning (criterion E). The disturbance is not due to the direct physiological effects of a substance (i.e., a drug of abuse, a medication, or toxin exposure) or a general medical condition and does not occur exclusively during a mood disorder, a psychotic disorder, or a pervasive developmental disorder (criterion F).

The intensity, duration, or frequency of the anxiety and worry is far out of proportion to the actual likelihood or impact of the feared event. The person finds it difficult to keep worrisome thoughts from interfering with attention to tasks at hand and has difficulty stopping the worry. Adults with generalized anxiety disorder often worry about everyday, routine life circumstances such as possible job responsibilities, finances, the health of family members, misfortune to their children, or minor matters (such as household chores, car repairs, or being late for appointments). Children with generalized anxiety disorder tend to worry excessively about their competence or the quality of their performance. During the course of the disorder, the focus of worry may shift from one concern to another.

## PREVALENCE
In a community sample, the 1-year prevalence rate for generalized anxiety disorder was approximately 3% and the lifetime prevalence rate was 5%. In anxiety disorder clinics, approximately 12% of the individuals present with generalized anxiety disorder.

## COURSE
Many individuals with generalized anxiety disorder report that they have felt anxious and nervous all of their lives. Although over half of those presenting for treatment report onset in childhood or adolescence, onset occurring after age 20 years is not uncommon. The course is chronic but fluctuating and often worsens during times of stress.

*Reprinted with permission and adapted from the Diagnostic and Statistical Manual of Mental Disorders, Fourth Edition, Text Revision, Copyright 2000. American Psychiatric Association.*

# DSM-IV Criteria for Separation Anxiety Disorder

The following is a list of the DSM-IV criteria for separation anxiety disorder:

A. Developmentally inappropriate and excessive anxiety concerning separation from home or from those to whom the individual is attached, as evidenced by 3 (or more) of the following:

  (1) Recurrent excessive distress when separation from home or major attachment figures occurs or is anticipated
  (2) Persistent and excessive worry about losing, or about possible harm befalling, major attachment figures
  (3) Persistent and excessive worry that an untoward event will lead to separation from a major attachment figure (e.g., getting lost or being kidnapped)
  (4) Persistent reluctance or refusal to go to school or elsewhere because of fear of separation
  (5) Persistently and excessively fearful or reluctant to be alone or without major attachment figures at home or without significant adults in other settings
  (6) Persistent reluctance or refusal to go to sleep without being near a major attachment figure or to sleep away from home
  (7) Repeated nightmares involving the theme of separation
  (8) Repeated complaints of physical symptoms (such as headaches, stomachaches, nausea, or vomiting) when separation from major attachment figures occurs or is anticipated

B. The duration of the disturbance is at least 4 weeks.

C. The onset is before age 18 years.

D. The disturbance causes clinically significant distress or impairment in social, academic (occupational), or other important areas of functioning.

E. The disturbance does not occur exclusively during the course of a pervasive developmental disorder, schizophrenia, or other psychotic disorder, and, in adolescents and adults, is not better accounted for by panic disorder with agoraphobia. Specify if:

## EARLY ONSET
 If onset occurs before age 6 years

## PREVALENCE
Separation anxiety disorder is not uncommon; prevalence estimates average about 4% in children and adolescence.

## COURSE
Separation anxiety disorder may develop after some life stress (e.g., the death of a relative or pet, a change of schools, a move). Onset may be as early as preschool age and may occur at any time before 18 years of age, but onset as late as adolescence is uncommon.

# DSM-IV Criteria for Acute Stress Disorder

## DIAGNOSTIC FEATURES
The essential feature of acute stress disorder is the development of characteristic anxiety, dissociative, and other symptoms that occur within 1 month after exposure to an extreme traumatic stressor.

## Diagnostic Criteria for Acute Stress Disorder

| |
|---|
| A. The person has been exposed to a traumatic event in which both of the following were present:<br>(1) The person experienced, witnessed, or was confronted with an event or events that involved actual or threatened death or serious injury, or a threat to the physical integrity of self or others.<br>(2) The person's response involved intense fear, helplessness, or honor. |
| B. Either while experiencing or after experiencing the distressing event, the individual has 3 (or more) of the following dissociative symptoms:<br>(1) A subjective sense of numbing, detachment, or absence of emotional responsiveness<br>(2) A reduction in awareness of his or her surroundings (e.g., "being in a daze")<br>(3) Derealization<br>(4) Depersonalization<br>(5) Dissociative amnesia (i.e., the inability to recall an important aspect of the trauma) |
| C. The traumatic event is persistently reexperienced in at least 1 of the following ways: recurrent images, thoughts, dreams, illusions, flashback episodes, or a sense of reliving the experience; or distress on exposure to reminders of the traumatic event. |
| D. Marked avoidance of stimuli that arouse recollections of the trauma (e.g., thoughts, feelings, conversations, activities, places, people) |
| E. Marked symptoms of anxiety or increased arousal (e.g., difficulty sleeping, irritability, poor concentration, hypervigilance, exaggerated startle response, motor restlessness) |
| F. The disturbance causes clinically significant distress or impairment in social, occupational, or other important areas of functioning or impairs the individual's ability to pursue some necessary task, such as obtaining necessary assistance or mobilizing personal resources by telling family members about the traumatic experience. |
| G. The disturbance lasts for a minimum of 2 days and a maximum of 4 weeks and occurs within 4 weeks of the traumatic event. |
| H. The disturbance is not due to the direct physiological effects of a substance (e.g., a drug of abuse, a medication) or a general medical condition, is not better accounted for by brief psychotic disorder, and is not merely an exacerbation of a preexisting Axis I or Axis II disorder. |

## PREVALENCE
The prevalence of acute stress disorder in a population exposed to a serious traumatic stress depends on the severity and persistence of the trauma and degree of exposure to it.

## COURSE
Symptoms of acute stress disorder are experienced during or immediately after the trauma, last for at least 2 days, and either resolve within 4 weeks after the conclusion of the traumatic event or the diagnosis is changed. When symptoms persist beyond 1 month, a diagnosis of posttraumatic stress disorder (PTSD) may be appropriate if the full criteria for PTSD are met. The severity, duration, and proximity of an individual's exposure to the traumatic event are the most important factors in determining the likelihood of development of acute stress disorder.

*Reprinted with permission and adapted from the Diagnostic and Statistical Manual of Mental Disorders, Fourth Edition, Text Revision, Copyright 2000. American Psychiatric Association.*

# DSM-IV Criteria for Posttraumatic Stress Disorder

## DIAGNOSTIC FEATURES

The essential feature of posttraumatic stress disorder (PTSD) is the development of characteristic symptoms following exposure to an extreme traumatic stressor involving direct personal experience of an event that involves actual or threatened death or serious injury, or other threat to one's physical integrity; or witnessing an event that involves death, injury, or a threat to the physical integrity of another person; or learning about unexpected or violent death, serious harm, or threat of death or injury experienced by a family member or other close associate.

## Diagnostic Criteria for PTSD

A. The person has been exposed to a traumatic event in which both of the following were present:
 (1) The person experienced, witnessed, or was confronted with an event or events that involved actual or threatened death or serious injury, or a threat to the physical integrity of self or others.
 (2) The person's response involved intense fear, helplessness, or horror.
 *Note:* In children, this may be expressed by disorganized or agitated behavior.

B. The traumatic event is persistently re-experienced in 1 (or more) of the following ways:
 (1) Recurrent and intrusive distressing recollections of the event, including images, thoughts, or perceptions
 *Note:* In young children, repetitive play may occur in which themes or aspects of the trauma are expressed.
 (2) Recurrent distressing dreams of the event
 *Note:* In children, there may be frightening dreams without recognizable content.
 (3) Acting or feeling as if the traumatic event were recurring (includes a sense of reliving the experience, illusions, hallucinations, and dissociative flashback episodes, including those that occur on awakening or when intoxicated). *Note:* In young children, trauma-specific reenactment may occur.
 (4) Intense psychological distress at exposure to internal or external cues that symbolize or resemble an aspect of the traumatic event
 (5) Physiological reactivity on exposure to internal or external cues that symbolize or resemble an aspect of the traumatic event

C. Persistent avoidance of stimuli associated with the trauma and numbing of general responsiveness (not present before the trauma), as indicated by 3 (or more) of the following:
 (1) Efforts to avoid thoughts, feelings, or conversations associated with the trauma
 (2) Efforts to avoid activities, places, or people that arouse recollections of the trauma
 (3) Inability to recall an important aspect of the trauma
 (4) Markedly diminished interest or participation in significant activities
 (5) Feeling of detachment or estrangement from others
 (6) Restricted range of affect (unable to have loving feelings)

| | |
|---|---|
| (7) Sense of a foreshortened future (e.g., does not expect to have a career, marriage, children, or a normal life span) | |

| | |
|---|---|
| D. | Persistent symptoms of increased arousal (not present before the trauma), as indicated by 2 (or more) of the following:<br>(1) Difficulty falling or staying asleep<br>(2) Irritability or outbursts of anger<br>(3) Difficulty concentrating<br>(4) Hypervigilance<br>(5) Exaggerated startle response |

| | |
|---|---|
| E. | Duration of the disturbance is more than 1 month. |

| | |
|---|---|
| F. | The disturbance causes clinically significant distress or impairment in social, occupational, or other important areas of functioning. |

*Specify if:*   **Acute:** if duration of symptoms is less than 3 months
             **Chronic:** if duration of symptoms is 3 months or more
             **With delayed onset:** if onset of symptoms is at least 6 months after the stressor

## PREVALENCE
Community-based studies reveal a lifetime prevalence for PTSD ranging from 1% to 14%. Studies of at-risk individuals (e.g., victims of criminal violence) have yielded prevalence rates ranging from 3 to 58%.

## COURSE
PTSD can occur at any age, including during childhood. Symptoms usually begin within the first 3 months of the trauma, although there may be a delay of months or even years before symptoms appear.

Frequently, the disturbance first meets criteria for acute stress disorder. Duration of the symptoms varies, with complete recovery occurring within 3 months in approximately half of the cases, with many others having persisting symptoms for longer than 12 months after the trauma.

# DSM-IV Criteria for Obsessive-Compulsive Disorder

## DIAGNOSTIC FEATURES

The essential features of obsessive-compulsive disorder are recurrent obsessions or compulsions that are severe enough to be time consuming (i.e., they take more than 1 hour a day to act out) or cause marked distress or significant impairment.

## Diagnostic Criteria for Obsessive-Compulsive Disorder (OCD)

<table>
<tr><td>

A. Either obsessions or compulsions:

Obsessions as defined by (1), (2), (3), and (4):

   (1) Recurrent and persistent thoughts, impulses, or images that are experienced, at some time during the disturbance, as intrusive and inappropriate and that cause marked anxiety or distress

   (2) The thoughts, impulses, or images are not simply excessive worries about real-life problems

   (3) The person attempts to ignore or suppress such thoughts, impulses, or images, or to neutralize them with some other thought or action

   (4) The person recognized that the obsessional thoughts, impulses, or images are a product of his or her own mind (not imposed from without as in thought insertion)

Compulsions as defined by (1) and (2):

   (1) Repetitive behaviors (e.g., hand washing, ordering, checking) or mental acts (e.g., praying, counting, repeating words silently) that the person feels driven to perform in response to an obsession, or according to rules that must be applied rigidly

   (2) The behaviors or mental acts are aimed at preventing or reducing distress or preventing some dreaded event or situation; however, these behaviors or mental acts either are not connected in a realistic way with what they are designed to neutralize or prevent or are clearly excessive

</td></tr>
<tr><td>

B. At some point during the course of the disorder, the person has recognized that the obsessions or compulsions are excessive or unreasonable. Note: This does not apply to children.

</td></tr>
<tr><td>

C. The obsessions or compulsions cause marked distress, are time consuming (take more than 1 hour a day to act out), or significantly interfere with the person's normal routine, occupational (or academic) functioning, or usual social activities or relationships.

</td></tr>
<tr><td>

D. If another Axis I disorder is present, the content of the obsessions or compulsions is not restricted to it (e.g., preoccupation with food in the presence of an eating disorder).

</td></tr>
<tr><td>

E. The disturbance is not due to the direct physiological effects of a substance (e.g., a drug of abuse, a medication) or a general medical condition.

</td></tr>
</table>

*Specify if:* With poor insight: If, for most of the time during the current episode, the person does not recognize that the obsessions and compulsions are excessive or unreasonable

## PREVALENCE

Recent community studies have estimated a lifetime prevalence of 1.5 to 2.1%.

## COURSE

Obsessive-compulsive disorder usually begins in adolescence, but it may begin in childhood. Modal age at onset is usually between the ages of 6 and 15 for males and between ages 20 and 29 for females. The majority of individuals have a chronic waxing and waning course, with exacerbation of symptoms that may be related to stress.

# DSM-IV Criteria for Panic Disorder without Agoraphobia

The following are a list of the criteria for panic disorder.

A.  Both (1) and (2):

  1.  Recurrent unexpected panic attacks
  2.  At least 1 of the attacks has been followed by 1 month (or more) of 1 (or more) of the following:

  Persistent concern about having additional attacks

  Worry about the implications of the attack or its consequences (e.g., losing control, having a heart attack, "going crazy")

  A significant change in behavior related to the attacks

B.  Absence of agoraphobia (i.e., anxiety about being in places or situations from which escape might be difficult or in which help may not be available in the event of having a panic attack; the anxiety typically leads to a pervasive avoidance of a variety of situations that may include being alone outside the home or being home alone; being in a crowd of people; traveling in an automobile, bus, or airplane; or being on a bridge or in an elevator)

C.  The panic attacks are not due to the direct physiological effects of a substance (e.g., a drug of abuse, a medication) or a general medical condition (e.g., hyperthyroidism).

D.  The panic attacks are not better accounted for by another mental disorder, such as social phobia (e.g., occurring on exposure to feared social situations), specific phobia (e.g., on exposure to a specific phobic situation), obsessive-compulsive disorder (e.g., on exposure to dirt in someone with an obsession about contamination), posttraumatic stress disorder (e.g., in response to stimuli associated with a severe stressor), or separation anxiety disorder (e.g., in response to being away from home or close relatives).

*Reprinted with permission and adapted from the Diagnostic and Statistical Manual of Mental Disorders, Fourth Edition, Text Revision, Copyright 2000. American Psychiatric Association.*

# DSM-IV Criteria for Panic Attack and Panic Disorder

## PANIC ATTACK

Panic attacks occur in the context of several different anxiety disorders. The essential feature of a panic attack is a discrete period of intense fear or discomfort that is accompanied by at least 4 of 13 somatic or cognitive symptoms. The attack has a sudden onset and builds to a peak rapidly (usually in 10 minutes or less) and is often accompanied by a sense of imminent danger or impending doom and an urge to escape.

### Criteria for Panic Attack

*Note:* A panic attack is not a codable disorder. Code the specific diagnosis in which the panic attack occurs (e.g., 300.01 panic disorder without agoraphobia).

A panic attack is defined as a discrete period of intense fear or discomfort, in which 4 (or more) of the following symptoms developed abruptly and reached a peak within 10 minutes:

(1)  Palpitations, pounding heart, or accelerated heart rate
(2)  Sweating
(3)  Trembling or shaking
(4)  Sensations of shortness of breath or smothering
(5)  Feeling of choking
(6)  Chest pain or discomfort
(7)  Nausea or abdominal distress
(8)  Feeling dizzy, unsteady, lightheaded, or faint
(9)  Derealization (feelings of unreality) or depersonalization (being detached from oneself)
(10) Fear of losing control or going crazy
(11) Fear of dying
(12) Paresthesias (numbness or tingling sensations)
(13) Chills or hot flashes

## PANIC DISORDER

The essential feature of panic disorder is the presence of recurrent, unexpected panic attacks followed by at least 1 month of persistent concern about having another panic attack, worry about the possible implications or consequences of the panic attacks, or a significant behavioral change related to the attacks (criterion A). The panic attacks are not due to the direct physiological effects of a substance (e.g., caffeine intoxication) or a general medical condition (e.g., hyperthyroidism) (criterion C). Finally, the panic attacks are not better accounted for by another mental disorder (e.g., specific or social phobia, obsessive-compulsive disorder, posttraumatic stress disorder, or separation anxiety disorder) (criterion B).

An unexpected (spontaneous, uncued) panic attack is defined as one that is not associated with a situational trigger (i.e., it occurs "out of the blue"). At least 2 unexpected panic attacks are required for the diagnosis, but most individuals have considerably more. Individuals with panic disorder frequently also have situationally predisposed panic attacks (i.e., those more likely to occur on, but not invariably associated with, exposure to a situational trigger). Situationally bound attacks (e.g., those that occur almost invariably and immediately on exposure to a situational trigger) can occur but are less common.

The frequency and severity of the panic attacks vary widely. For example, some individuals have moderately frequent attacks (e.g., once a week) that occur regularly for months at a time. Others report short bursts of more frequent attacks (e.g., daily for a week) separated by weeks or months without any attacks or with less frequent attacks (e.g., 2 each month) over many years. Limited-symptom attacks (i.e., attacks that are identical to "full" panic attacks except that the sudden fear or anxiety is accompanied by fewer than 4 of the 13 additional symptoms) are very common in individuals with panic disorder. Although the distinction between full panic attacks and limited-symptom attacks is somewhat arbitrary, full panic attacks are associated with greater morbidity. Most individuals who have limited-symptom attacks have full panic attacks at some time during the course of the disorder.

Individuals with panic disorder display characteristic concerns or attributions about the implications or consequences of the panic attacks. Some fear that the attacks indicate the presence of an undiagnosed, life-threatening illness (e.g., cardiac diseases, seizure disorder). Despite repeated medical testing and reassurance, they may remain frightened and unconvinced that they do not have a life-threatening illness. Others fear that the panic attacks are an indication that they are "going crazy" or losing control or are emotionally weak. Some individuals with recurrent panic attacks significantly change their behavior (e.g., quit a job) in response to the attacks, but deny either fear of having another attack or concerns about the consequences of their panic attacks. Concerns about the next attack, or its implications, are often associated with development of avoidant behavior that may meet criteria for agoraphobia, in which case panic disorder with agoraphobia is diagnosed.

## PREVALENCE

Epidemiological studies throughout the world consistently indicate the lifetime prevalence of panic disorder (with or without agoraphobia) to be between 1.5 and 3.5%. One-year prevalence rates are between 1 and 2%. Approximately one third to one half of individuals diagnosed with panic disorder in community samples also have agoraphobia, although a much higher rate of agoraphobia is encountered in clinical samples.

## COURSE

Age at onset of panic disorder varies considerably, but is most typically between late adolescence and the mid-30s. There may be a bimodal distribution, with one peak in late adolescence and a second, smaller peak in the mid-30s. A small number of cases begin in childhood, and onset after age 45 years is unusual but can occur. Retrospective descriptions by individuals seen in clinical settings suggest that the usual course is chronic but waxing and waning. Some individuals may have episodic outbreaks with years of remission in between, and others may have continuous severe symptomatology. Although agoraphobia may develop at any point, its onset is usually within the first year of occurrence of recurrent panic attacks. The course of agoraphobia and its relationship to the course of panic attacks are variable. In some cases, a decrease or remission of panic attacks may be followed closely by a corresponding decrease in agoraphobic avoidance and anxiety. In others, agoraphobia may become chronic regardless of the presence or absence of panic attacks by avoiding certain situations. Naturalistic follow-up studies of individuals treated in tertiary care settings (which may select for a poor-prognosis group) suggest that, at 6-10 years post-treatment, about 30% of individuals are well, 40-50% are improved but symptomatic, and the remaining 20-30% have symptoms that are the same or slightly worse.

# Screening Tools for Anxiety in Children/Teens

## The State-Trait Anxiety Inventory for Children
## (Charles D. Spielberger, C.D. Edwards, J. Montuori & R. Lushene)

### Description of the State-Trait Anxiety Inventory for Children (STAIC)

The STAIC differentiates between proneness to anxious behavior rooted in personality (trait anxiety) and anxiety as a fleeting emotional state (state anxiety). The instrument is targeted to measure anxiety in upper elementary or junior high school students. It consists of two 20-item Likert scales. The separate, self-report scales are designed to measure two distinct anxiety concepts: state anxiety (S-Anxiety) and trait anxiety (T-Anxiety).

The STAIC S-Anxiety scale consists of 20 statements that ask children how they feel at a *particular moment in time*. Examples from the **STAIC S-Anxiety** questionnaire include:

| 1. I feel | very relaxed | relaxed | not relaxed |
|-----------|--------------|---------|-------------|
| 2. I feel | very upset | upset | not upset |

The STAIC T-Anxiety scale also consists of 20 item statements, but children respond to these items by indicating how they *generally* feel. Examples from the **STAIC T-Anxiety** questionnaire include:

| 1. I worry too much | hardly ever | sometimes | often |
|---------------------|-------------|-----------|-------|
| 2. I notice my heart beats fast | hardly ever | sometimes | often |

### Age Range

While especially constructed to measure anxiety in 9- to 12-year-old children, the STAIC also may be used for younger children with average or above reading ability and for older children who are below average in ability.

### Psychometric Properties of the STAIC

Studies have supported the validity and internal consistency of the STAIC. Normed scores are available for fourth-, fifth-, and sixth-grade elementary school children.

### Ordering Information:

©1973. The tool can be ordered online from Mind Garden at www.mindgarden.com/ or by calling 650-261-3550.
The State-Trait Anxiety Inventory for Adults (Charles D. Spielberger, R.L. Gorsuch & R.E. Lushene, R. E.)

# The State-Trait Anxiety Inventory for Adults
## (Charles D. Spielberger, R.L. Gorsuch & R.E. Lushene, R.E.)

## Description of the State-Trait Anxiety Inventory (STAI)

The STAI is used to measure anxiety in adults. The STAI clearly differentiates between the temporary condition of "state anxiety" and the more general and long-standing quality of "trait anxiety." The essential qualities evaluated by the STAIS-Anxiety scale are feelings of apprehension, tension, nervousness, and worry. Scores on the STAIS-Anxiety scale increase in response to physical danger and psychological stress, and decrease as a result of relaxation training. On the STAIT-Anxiety scale, consistent with the trait anxiety construct, psychoneurotic and depressed patients generally have high scores. The STAI consists of two 20-item Likert scales and can be administered in 10 minutes.

The S-Anxiety scale consists of twenty statements that evaluate how respondents feel "right now, at this moment." Examples from the STAIS-Anxiety scale include:

| A. I feel at ease | 0 | 1 | 2 | 3 |
|---|---|---|---|---|
| B. I feel upset | 0 | 1 | 2 | 3 |

*Scale: 0 = Not at all, 1 = Somewhat, 2 = Moderately so, 3 = Very much so*

The T-Anxiety scale consists of twenty statements that assess how respondents feel "generally." Examples from the STAIT-Anxiety scale include:

| A. I am a steady person | 1 | 2 | 3 | 4 |
|---|---|---|---|---|
| B. I lack self-confidence | 1 | 2 | 3 | 4 |

*Scale: 1 =Almost never, 2 = Sometimes, 3 = Often, 4=Almost Always*

## Age Range

Adults as well as high-school and college-age students, with norm groups of high school, college, 19-39 years old, 40-49 years old, 50-69 years old

## Psychometric Properties

The STAI is a valid and highly reliable tool for measuring anxiety. Normed scores are available for adults as well as for high school and college students.

## Ordering Information:

©1970. It can be ordered online from Mind Garden at www.mindgarden.com/ or by calling 650-261-3550.

# KySS Worries Questionnaire (Ages 10-21 years)
## (B. Melnyk and Z. Moldenhauer)

## Description of the KySS Worries Questionnaire

The KySS Worries Questionnaire is a 15 item Likert-scale questionnaire that taps common worries in older school-age children and youth. A parent version of the scale also is available. The original scale consisted of 13 items. Two additional items (#14-weight and #15-level of activity/exercise) have recently been added to the scale.

## Age Range

The worries questionnaire is targeted for use with older school-age children and teens, between the ages of 10 and 21 years of age. A separate scale targets the worries of parents of school-age children and teens.

## Psychometric Properties

Content validity was established by pediatric and mental health experts. Face validity was established by 15 parents as well as 15 children and teens, between 10 and 20 years of age. Cronbach's alpha with a sample of 621 school-age children and teens was .87 for the first 13 items on the scale. Cronbach's alpha with a sample of 603 parents was .90 for the first 13 items on the scale.

# KySS Worries Questionnaire (Ages 10-21 years)
## (B. Melnyk and Z. Moldenhauer)

**Please answer each of the following questions by circling your answers.**

Do you worry about any of the following for yourself?

|  |  | Not at all | Sometimes always | Often | Nearly | Always |
|---|---|---|---|---|---|---|
| 1) | Depression | 1 | 2 | 3 | 4 | 5 |
| 2) | Anxiety | 1 | 2 | 3 | 4 | 5 |
| 3) | Parents separating or divorcing | 1 | 2 | 3 | 4 | 5 |
| 4) | Violence/being hurt | 1 | 2 | 3 | 4 | 5 |
| 5) | Physical abuse/neglect | 1 | 2 | 3 | 4 | 5 |
| 6) | Sexual abuse/rape | 1 | 2 | 3 | 4 | 5 |
| 7) | Sexual activity | 1 | 2 | 3 | 4 | 5 |
| 8) | Substance abuse | 1 | 2 | 3 | 4 | 5 |
| 9) | Eating disorders | 1 | 2 | 3 | 4 | 5 |
| 10) | Problems with your self-esteem | 1 | 2 | 3 | 4 | 5 |
| 11) | Your relationship with your parents | 1 | 2 | 3 | 4 | 5 |
| 12) | Knowing how to cope with things that stress you | 1 | 2 | 3 | 4 | 5 |
| 13) | Being made fun of by your friends | 1 | 2 | 3 | 4 | 5 |
| 14) | Your weight | 1 | 2 | 3 | 4 | 5 |
| 15) | Your level of activity/exercise | 1 | 2 | 3 | 4 | 5 |

16) Do you have any other worries? If yes, please describe them.

_____

_____

17) Do your worries interfere with your ability to do school work?     ___ Yes ___No

18) Do your worries affect your relationship with your friends?     ___ Yes ___ No

# KySS Worries Questionnaire for Parents
## (B. Melnyk and Z. Moldenhauer)

**Please answer each of the following questions by circling your answers.**

Do you worry about any of the following for your child?

| | | Not at all | Sometimes | Often | Nearly always | Always |
|---|---|---|---|---|---|---|
| 1) | Depression | 1 | 2 | 3 | 4 | 5 |
| 2) | Anxiety | 1 | 2 | 3 | 4 | 5 |
| 3) | Parents separating or divorcing | 1 | 2 | 3 | 4 | 5 |
| 4) | Violence/being hurt | 1 | 2 | 3 | 4 | 5 |
| 5) | Physical abuse/neglect | 1 | 2 | 3 | 4 | 5 |
| 6) | Sexual abuse/rape | 1 | 2 | 3 | 4 | 5 |
| 7) | Sexual activity | 1 | 2 | 3 | 4 | 5 |
| 8) | Substance abuse | 1 | 2 | 3 | 4 | 5 |
| 9) | Eating disorders | 1 | 2 | 3 | 4 | 5 |
| 10) | Self-esteem | 1 | 2 | 3 | 4 | 5 |
| 11) | Your relationship with your child | 1 | 2 | 3 | 4 | 5 |
| 12) | How your child copes with stressful things | 1 | 2 | 3 | 4 | 5 |
| 13) | Being "bullied" by classmates | 1 | 2 | 3 | 4 | 5 |
| 14) | Your child's weight | 1 | 2 | 3 | 4 | 5 |
| 15) | Your child's level of activity/exercise | 1 | 2 | 3 | 4 | 5 |

16)     Do you have any other worries about your child? If yes, please describe them.



17)     Do your child's worries interfere with his/ her ability to do school work? __Yes __No

18)     Do your child's worries interfere with his or her friendships? ___ Yes ___ No

# Information for Parents about Anxiety in Children and Teens

## Quick Facts

- Fear and anxiety are a normal part of growing up, but they should not interfere with your child's daily activities.
- Anxiety disorders are among the most common mental health problems in children and teens.
- Children and teens with anxiety experience severe and persistent distress that interferes with their daily functioning; often these disorders are under-diagnosed.
- You might describe your child as a "worrier."
- Children and teens will often report physical complaints or describe "feeling sick" (e.g. stomach pain, headaches, chest pain, and fatigue).
- Many times, children with anxiety also are having problems with paying attention/staying focused at school; they may have problems being "moody."
- Many times, healthcare providers will mistake anxiety symptoms for attention deficit symptoms.

## Common Signs of Anxiety for Kids and Teens:

| Physical | Behavioral | Thoughts |
|---|---|---|
| Restlessness and irritability(very common in younger children) Headaches Stomachaches, nausea, vomiting, diarrhea Feeling tired Palpitations, increased heart rate, increased blood pressure Hyperventilation/shortness of breath Muscle tension Difficulty sleeping Dizziness, tingling fingers, weakness Tremors | Escape/avoidant behaviors Crying Clinging to/fear of separating from parents Speaking in a soft voice Variations in speech patterns Nail-biting Thumb-sucking Always "checking out" surroundings Freezing Regression (bedwetting, temper tantrums) | Worry about "what ifs…" Always thinking something terrible will happen Unreasonable, rigid thinking |

## Medical Problems That Mimic Anxiety Symptoms

- Low blood sugar
- Thyroid problems
- Seizures

- Irregular heart beat
- Migraine headaches
- Breathing problems

## Medications/Drugs That May Cause Anxiety Symptoms

- Caffeine
- Nicotine
- Antihistamines (Benadryl)
- Medications for asthma
- Marijuana
- Nasal decongestants, such as pseudoephedrine
- Stimulant medications (e.g., Ritalin)
- Street drugs (e.g., cocaine)
- Steroids
- Prescribed medications to treat anxiety, when started, can cause effects that mimic anxiety symptoms, but these symptoms often subside after a few days.

## Treatment

- Talk to your primary care provider if you have concerns; describe what you are noticing about your child.
- Ask your primary care provider for things to read or Web sites to visit to learn more about your child's symptoms.
- Therapy might be recommended to help treat your child's symptoms. It could involve individual, group, or family work.
- Consider what could be changed at home or in school to help your child deal with his or her worries (e.g., set a regular bedtime routine or think about which activities are stressful for your child and think about ways to handle them differently).
- Medication is often recommended as an alternative treatment if symptoms are disturbing your child's day-to-day activities. Your provider may recommend a class of medicines called "SSRIs, short for Selective Serotonin Reuptake Inhibitors."
- Be sure to ask:
  - What symptoms will the medication treat?
  - How long will my child have to take this medication?
  - How much medication will my child have to take, and how many times a day will he/she have to take it?
  - What happens if my child misses a dose of medication?
  - How do we stop the medication?

# Information for Parents on How to Help Your Child/Teen Cope with Stressful Events or Uncertainty

The most important thing that you can do to help your child/teen cope with stressful events is to remain as calm as possible when you are with him or her. Children pick up on their parents' anxiety very quickly. If they sense you are anxious, they will be anxious as well. Therefore, if you are having difficulty coping with a stressful situation, it is a good idea to reach out to resources to help yourself, such as friends, family members, support groups, clergy, or healthcare professionals. Taking care of your own stress so that you are less anxious will help your child to stay calm.

## Recognize Signs of Anxiety/Stress in Your Child

- Children and teens typically regress when stressed. That is, they go back to doing things they did when they were younger to help themselves feel more comfortable and secure. For instance, a preschool child may go back to sucking his/her thumb and a school-age child or teen may act more dependent upon their parents or have difficulty separating from them.

- Other common signs of anxiety in young children include: restlessness/hyperactivity, temper tantrums, nightmares, clinging behaviors, difficulty separating, and distress around new people.

- Common signs of anxiety in older school age-children and teens include: difficulty concentrating and sleeping, anger, restlessness/hyperactivity, worry, and physical complaints, such as stomachaches or headaches.

- At age 9 years, children realize that death is permanent. Fears of death or physical violence and harm are often common after this age.

- Signs and symptoms of anxiety such as these are usually healthy, temporary coping strategies that help your child to deal with stress. However, if these symptoms persist for several weeks or interfere with your child's functioning, talk to your child's primary healthcare provider about them. Your child's doctor or nurse practitioner will know what to do to help.

- Be honest and give age-appropriate and developmentally appropriate explanations about stressful events when they occur.

- For young children (under 8 years of age), only provide answers to questions they are asking and do not overwhelm them with too much detail. Use language that young children can understand. Do not expose young children to visual images in the newspapers or on television that may be terrifying.

- It may be easier for young children to express how they are feeling by asking them to talk about how their stuffed animals or dolls are feeling or thinking.

- Help children and teens to express how they are feeling about what they have seen or heard. If children have difficulty verbally expressing their feelings, ask them to make a drawing about how they are feeling. Older school-age children and teens can benefit from writing about how they feel.

- Ask your child/teen, "What is the scariest or worst thing about this event for you?" or "What is worrying you the most right now?" and take time to really listen to what he or she has to say.

- Reassure children that they did nothing wrong to cause what happened. Toddlers and preschool children, especially, feel guilty when stressful events happen.

- Tell children and teens that what they are feeling (e.g., anger, anxiety, and helplessness) is normal and that others feel the same way.

- Decrease anxiety in your child by reassuring him or her that you will get through this together. Emphasize that adults are doing everything possible to take care of the stressful situation and that he or she is not alone.

- Help your child/teen to release tension by encouraging daily physical exercise and activities.

- Continue to provide as much structure to your child's schedules and days as possible.

- Recognize that added stress/anxiety usually increases psychological or physical symptoms (e.g., headaches or abdominal pain) in children/teens that are already anxious or depressed.

- Young children who are depressed typically have different symptoms (e.g., restlessness, excessive motor activity) from those experienced by older school-age children or teens who are depressed (e.g., sad or withdrawn affect; anger, difficulty sleeping or eating; talking about feeling hopeless).

- Use this opportunity as a time to work with your child on their coping skills (e.g., relaxation techniques, positive reappraisal, and prayer). Children watch how their parents cope and often take on the same coping strategies. Therefore, showing your child that you use positive coping strategies to deal with stress will help him or her to develop healthy ways of coping.

- Be sure to have your child or teen seen by a healthcare provider or mental health professional for signs or symptoms of persistent anxiety, depression, recurrent pain, persistent behavioral changes, or if he or she has difficulty maintaining routine schedules.

- Remember that stressful times can be an opportunity to build future coping and life skills as well as to bring your family closer together.

# Information for Helping Children, Teens, and Their Families Cope with War and/or Terrorism

1. Be honest and give age-appropriate and developmentally appropriate explanations about the traumatic event.

   - For young children, in particular, only provide answers to questions they are asking and do not overwhelm them with too much detail.

   - Use language that young children can understand.

   - It may be easier for young children to express how they are feeling by asking them to talk about how their stuffed animals or dolls are feeling or thinking.

   - Help children and teens to express how they are feeling about what they have seen or heard. If children have difficulty verbally expressing their feelings, ask them to make a drawing about how they are feeling. Older school-age children and teens can benefit from writing about how they feel.

   - Ask children and teens, "What is the scariest or worst thing about this for you?" or "What is worrying you the most?"

2. Do not expose young children to visual images in the newspapers or on television that are potentially terrifying.

3. Reassure children that they did nothing wrong to cause what happened.

   - Toddlers and preschool children, especially, feel guilty when something tragic happens.

4. Tell children and teens that what they are feeling (e.g., anger, anxiety, and helplessness) is normal and that others feel the same way.

5. Alleviate some of their anxiety by reassuring children that we will get through this together and will be stronger as a result of what we have been through. Emphasize that adults will be there to help them through this and that they are not alone.

6. Spend some special time with your child every day, even if only 15 minutes.

7. Help children and teens to release their tension by encouraging daily physical exercise and activities.

8. Continue to provide structure to children's schedules and days.

9. Recognize that war or a tragic event could elevate psychological or physical symptoms (e.g., headaches, abdominal pain or chest pain, nightmares), especially in children and teens who are already depressed or anxious.

   • Remember that young children who are depressed typically have different symptoms (e.g., restlessness, excessive motor activity) from those experienced by older school-age children or teens who are depressed (e.g., sad or withdrawn affect; difficulty sleeping or eating; talking about feeling hopeless).

   • Anger can be a sign of anxiety in children and teens.

   • Children, even teens, who are stressed typically regress (e.g., revert to doing things that they did when they were younger, such as sucking their thumbs, bedwetting, or acting dependent upon their parents). This is a healthy temporary coping strategy. However, if these symptoms persist for several weeks, talk to your healthcare provider about them.

10. Use this opportunity as a time to work with children on their coping skills.

    • Use coping strategies that you know are typically helpful for your child, since each child copes in a way that is best for him or her (e.g., prayer, doing things to help other people, listening to music).

11. As a parent, remember that emotions are contagious. If you are highly upset or anxious, there is a good chance that your child also will feel the same way. If you are having difficulty coping with stress or with what is going on in the world around you, it is important to talk with someone who can help you to cope. You being calm will help your child to stay calm.

12. Be sure to have your child or teen seen by a healthcare provider or mental health professional for signs or symptoms of depression, persistent anxiety, recurrent pain, persistent behavioral changes, or if he or she has difficulty maintaining routine schedules.

13. Remember that this can be an opportunity to build future coping and life skills as well as to bring your family unit closer together.

# Information for Teens and School-Age Children about Stress and Anxiety

## Quick Facts
- It is common for older children and teens to struggle with feelings of anxiety or stress and to worry about things (real or made up).
- These feelings can make it hard to go to school, talk with teachers, or hang out with friends.
- Your parents, teachers, and friends might describe you as a "worrier".
- Your body feels worry too. You might not feel good and may have headaches, stomachaches, or feel tired, especially when you have to do something that stresses you.
- Worry can make it hard to pay attention at school. It can even make you feel sad, angry/grumpy, or frustrated!
- Most people, at some time in their lives, need help to deal with stress. There is nothing to be ashamed of in asking for help with how you feel.
- There are many things you can do to help feel less stressed and worried.
- It is important to see a doctor or practitioner to talk about your worries and to undergo a check-up, as it is important to make sure that there is not a medical reason for why you are feeling the way that you do.

## What You Can Do About Worry and Stress
- Talk to someone you trust about how you are feeling.
- If you have trouble talking, write down how you feel and then share it with someone.
- Try to do relaxing exercises (imagine being at your favorite place; take slow deep breaths and, when you breathe out, imagine all of your stress leaving you; listen to calming music).
- Do positive self-talk (e.g., "I am feeling calmer; I am going to handle this well").
- Stay focused in the present moment (try not to feel guilty about something that has happened in the past or worry about the future, because most things we worry about don't ever happen).
- Exercise for at least 30 minutes 3 to 4 days a week (this is a great way to release stress!).
- Don't take certain medications or drugs that can cause you to feel anxiety.
  These include caffeine, which is found in Pepsi, Mountain Dew, coffee, and tea; nicotine in cigarettes; marijuana; nasal decongestants (e.g., Sudafed); stimulant medication (e.g. Ritalin), or street drugs (e.g. cocaine).

## When What You Are Doing Isn't Helping
- Talk to your parent(s), your doctor, or nurse practitioner if you think you worry too much about things. Describe how you think and feel.
- Ask your primary care provider for things to read or Web sites to visit so you and your parents can learn more about how you are feeling.
- Your doctor or practitioner might want you to meet with a counselor to help you with your worries. You might meet with the counselor alone, with your family, or in a group with other kids who have the same problems.
- Medication may help to stop your worry. Ask your doctor or practitioner how this could help.

# Internet Resources

## American Academy of Child and Adolescent Psychiatry
www.aacap.org
This Web site is an excellent source of information on the assessment and treatment of child and adolescent mental health disorders. Handouts for use with families (i.e., *Facts for Families*) are available on a multitude of problems, including anxiety disorders.

## KidsHealth
www.kidshealth.org
This is an outstanding Web site that contains health information for healthcare providers, parents, teens, and children. Many of the topics relate to emotions and behaviors (e.g., anxiety, fears, depression) and are developmentally sensitive to specific age groups. Physicians and other healthcare providers review all material before it is posted on this Web site.

## National Association of Pediatric Nurse Practitioners' (NAPNAP) KySS Program
www.napnap.org
This site can be accessed to keep abreast of all ongoing and new initiatives of the KySS Program. Some handouts for downloading and use in practice are available to assist families in dealing with stressful situations (e.g., war, terrorism).

# References

American Psychiatric Association (2000). *Diagnostic and Statistical Manual of Mental Disorders, Fourth Edition* (DSM-IV). Washington, D.C.: APA.

Kaye, D.L., Montgomery, M.E., & Munson, S. (2002). *Child and Adolescent Mental Health.* Philadelphia, Pa: Lippincott.

Jellinek, M., Patel, B.P., & Froehle, M. (2002). *Bright Futures in Practice: Mental Health- Vol I. Practice Guide.* Arlington, VA: National Center for Education in Maternal and Child Health.

Jellinek, M., Patel, B.P. & Froehle, M. (2002). *Bright Futures in Practice: Mental Health- Vol II. Tool Kit.* Arlington, VA: National Center for Education in Maternal and Child Health.

Melnyk, B.M., Brown, H., Jones, D.C., Kreipe, R., & Novak, J. (2003). Improving the mental/psychosocial health of U.S. children and adolescents. Outcomes and implementation strategies from the national KySS summit. *Journal of Pediatric Health Care,* 17 (6) Supplement: S1-S24.

Moldenhauer, Z. & Melnyk, B.M. (in press for 2006). Assessment and management of common mental health disorders in children and adolescents. In N. Ryan-Wenger (Ed), NAPNAP/AFPNP: Core Curriculum for Pediatric Nurse Practitioners. Philadelphia, PA: Elsevier

## Information for Healthcare Providers about ADHD

### Quick Facts

ADHD is the most common behavior disorder in children.
ADHD is present in 4-12% of school-age children.
ADHD is more common in males than in females (3-6:1).
It typically presents during early childhood, before 7 years of age.
The disorder involves a persistent pattern of inattention, impulsiveness, or both.
Children with ADHD often have co-morbid disorders (e.g., anxiety disorders, learning disorders, oppositional defiant disorder).

### Co-morbidities Important for Assessment

Specific learning disabilities (10-40%)
Oppositional defiant disorder (30-60%)
Depression/anxiety disorders
Bipolar disorder
Fetal alcohol syndrome
Tourette's disorder
Psychosocial morbidities

### Mimics of ADHD

Language disorder
Learning disability
Anxiety/obsessive compulsive disorder
Depressive and bipolar disorders
Oppositional defiant disorder
Iron deficiency anemia
Malnutrition
Side effects of medication

Substance abuse
Sleep disorder
Child abuse/neglect
Stressful home environment
Parenting problem
Parental psychopathology
Inadequate educational setting

## Medical Conditions Associated With ADHD

Seizure disorder
Thyroid disorder
Traumatic brain injury
Fetal alcohol syndrome
Lead poisoning

## Testing that must be considered

Vision
Hearing
CBC with differential (to rule out anemia)
TSH, FT4 (to rule out thyroid disorders)
Lead screen
Genetic screen
Toxicology screen

## Rating Scales

Rating scales (e.g., the Vanderbilt; the Clinical Attention Profile) can be a useful adjunct in the diagnosis of ADHD and in the monitoring of response to treatment. Other helpful tools for ADHD can be downloaded as part of the National Initiative for Children's Healthcare Quality and the American Academy of Pediatrics' toolkit at www.nichq.org/resources/toolkit.

## Multiple Sources of Information

Information from parents, the child, teachers, primary care providers, and other caretakers is important for diagnostic consideration.

## Referral and Collaboration

It is important to refer a child with ADHD to a mental health provider when the condition has not improved in 3 months or if other co-morbid conditions exist (e.g., anxiety disorder, oppositional defiant disorder).

## Psycho-education and Follow-up/Pharmacotherapy

Psycho-education with the child, parents, and teachers is important as part of the management strategy. Careful follow-up is imperative, especially in monitoring initial response to medication therapy. Please see table 4.1 for pharmacotherapy treatment of ADHD.

# TABLE 4.1  Pharmacotherapy Treatment of Children and Adolescents with ADHD: Initial Dose, Kinetics, and Side Effects

| Drug | Dose | Kinetics | Side Effects/Comments |
|---|---|---|---|
| Methylphenidate HCl - short acting (*Ritalin/Methylin*) 5-, 10-, 20-mg tablets | Start: 0.3 mg/kg/dose or 2.5-5 mg before 8:00 AM and 12:00 noon. May increase by 0.1 mg/kg/dose weekly up to 0.3 - until 1.0 mg/kg/dose is reached. Maximum dose is 2 mg/kg/24 hrs or 80 mg/24 hrs. Not recommended for children < 5 years. | Onset: 30 min Peak: 1.9 hrs Duration: 4-6 hrs | Nervousness, insomnia, anorexia, weight loss, decreased height velocity, tics, stomachaches, headaches. Use with caution with underlying seizure disorder. Contraindicated: monoamine oxidase inhibitors. Monitor height, weight, blood pressure. Avoid caffeine and decongestants. Avoid doses after 4:00 PM. Consider drug holidays. |
| Methylphenidate HCl - intermediate acting (*Ritalin*-SR, *Metadate* ER, *Methylin* ER) 10-, 20-mg tablets | Starting dose 10 mg QD Maximum dose: 80 mg/day | Onset: 30-90 min Peak: 4.7 hrs Duration: 8 hrs | Do not crush or chew tablets. See comments for methylphenidate. |
| Methylphenidate HCl - long acting (*Metadate* CD, 20-mg tablets) (*Concerta*, 18-, 36-, 54-mg tablets) | Starting dose: 20 mg QD or 18 mg for *Concerta* Maximum dose: 80 mg/day of *Metadate* or 54 mg/day of *Concerta* | Onset: 30-90 min Peak: 4.7 hrs Duration: 8-12 hrs | Do not crush or chew tablets. See comments for methylphenidate. |
| Dextroamphetamine - short acting (*Dexedrine, Dextrostat*) 5-, 10-, 15-mg tablets, 5mg/mL elixir | 3-5 years: 2.5 mg/24 hrs every morning. Increase by 2.5 mg/24 hrs weekly. ≥ 6 yrs: 5 mg/24 hrs every morning. Increase by 5 mg/24 hrs at weekly intervals. Maximum dose: 40 mg/24 hrs. | Onset: 20 - 60 minutes Peak: 2 hrs Duration: 4-6 hrs | See comments for methylphenidate. Medication should generally not be used < 5 yrs because ADHD diagnosis should be made only with specialist consultation. |
| Dextroamphetamine - intermediate acting (*Adderall, Dexedrine Spansule*) 5-, 10-, 15-, 20-mg tablets, | 3-5 years: 2.5-5 mg QD or 0.3 mg/kg/dose. Increase by 2.5-5 mg every week. ≥ 6 years: 5 mg/24 hrs QD or 0.3 mg/kg/dose. Maximum dose: 40 mg/24 hrs. | Onset: 30-90 minutes Peak: 6-8 hrs | See comments for methylphenidate. |
| Dextroamphetamine - long acting (*Adderall* XR) | ≥ 6 years Starting dose: 5 mg QD or 0.3 mg/kg/dose. Maximum dose: 40 mg/24 hrs. | Onset: 30-90 min Duration: > 8 hrs | Limited information available. |

*Note:* Stimulants work best when given regularly. Adjust dose of stimulant medication as the child grows. There is a risk of abuse with stimulants.

*Caution:* Use stimulants cautiously in children with marked anxiety, tension, or agitation since these symptoms may be aggravated. Stimulants are contraindicated in children with motor tics or with a family history of diagnosis of Tourette's syndrome, although comorbid diagnosis of ADHD and Tourette's syndrome is rare. Avoid giving nasal decongestants with stimulants.

**Adapted from:**
- Green, S.M. (Ed.) (2003). Tarascon Pocket Pharmacopoeia Deluxe Download. Lompoc, Calif: Tarascon Publishing.
- *Robertson, J., & Shikofski, N. (Eds.) (2005).* Harriet Lane Handbook: A Manual for Pediatric House Officers *(17th Edition). St. Louis, MO: C.V. Mosby.*
- *Werry, J. S. & Aman, M.G. (Eds.) (1998).* Practitioner's Guide to Psychoactive Drugs for Children and Adolescents *(2nd Edition), New York, NY: Plenum Publishing Corporation.*

# DSM-IV Criteria for ADHD

Although most children have symptoms of inattention and hyperactivity/ impulsivity, there are some who display a predominant pattern of one or the other.

| |
|---|
| **I. Either A or B** |
| A. Six or more of the following symptoms of inattention have been present **for at least 6 months** to a point that is disruptive and inappropriate for developmental level: |
| **A. Inattention**<br><br>1. Often does not give close attention to details or makes careless mistakes in schoolwork, work, or other activities.<br>2. Often has trouble keeping attention on tasks or play activities.<br>3. Often does not seem to listen when spoken to directly.<br>4. Often does not follow instructions and fails to finish schoolwork, chores, or duties in the workplace (not due to oppositional behavior or failure to understand instructions).<br>5. Often have trouble organizing activities.<br>6. Often avoids, dislikes, or doesn't want to do things that take a lot of mental effort for a long period of time (such as schoolwork or homework).<br>7. Often loses things needed for tasks and activities (e.g., toys, school assignments, pencils, books, or tools).<br>8. Is often easily distracted.<br>9. Is often forgetful in daily activities. |
| B. Six or more of the following symptoms of hyperactivity-impulsivity have been present **for at least 6 months** to an extent that is disruptive and inappropriate for developmental level: |
| **B. Hyperactivity**<br><br>1. Often fidgets with hands or feet or squirms in seat.<br>2. Often gets up from seat when remaining in seat is expected.<br>3. Often runs about or climbs when and where it is not appropriate (adolescents or adults may feel very restless).<br>4. Often has trouble playing or enjoying leisure activities quietly.<br>5. Is often "on the go" or often acts as if "driven by a motor."<br>6. Often talks excessively. |

## Impulsivity

1. Often blurts out answers before questions have been finished.
2. Often has trouble waiting one's turn.
3. Often interrupts or intrudes on others (e.g., butts into conversations or games).
   II. Some symptoms that cause impairment were present before age 7 years.
   III. Some impairment from the symptoms is present in 2 or more settings (e.g., at school/work and at home).
   IV. There must be clear evidence of significant impairment in social, school, or work functioning.
   V. The symptoms do not happen only during the course of a pervasive developmental disorder, schizophrenia, or other psychotic disorder. The symptoms are not better accounted for by another mental disorder (e.g., mood disorder, anxiety disorder, dissociative disorder, or a personality disorder).

## Based on these criteria, 3 types of ADHD are identified

1. Combined Type: if both criteria 1A and 1B are met for the past 6 months
2. Predominantly Inattentive Type: if criterion 1A is met but criterion 1B is not met for the past 6 months
3. Predominantly Hyperactive-Impulsive Type: if criterion 1B is met but criterion 1A is not met for the past 6 months.

*Reprinted with permission and adapted from the Diagnostic and Statistical Manual of Mental Disorders, Fourth Edition, Text Revision, Copyright 2000. American Psychiatric Association.*

# Screening Tools for ADHD

## The National Initiative for Children's Healthcare Quality (NICHQ) Vanderbilt Assessment Scale for ADHD-Teacher as Initial Informant (M. Wolraich , et al)

### Description

The National Initiative for Children's Healthcare Quality (NICHQ) and American Academy of Pediatrics (AAP) have sponsored a set of tools for evaluating children with ADHD developed at Vanderbilt University. The initial evaluation scale monitors 43 symptoms for ADHD and other disorders and school performance as reported by a teacher.

### Parameters

(1) Symptoms (35)

(2) Performance (8) - academic (3) and classroom behavioral (5)

### Symptoms

(1) Fails to give attention to details or makes careless mistakes in schoolwork

(2) Has difficulty sustaining attention to tasks or activities

(3) Does not seem to listen when spoken to directly

(4) Does not follow through on instructions and fails to finish schoolwork (not due to oppositional behavior or failure to misunderstand)

(5) Has difficulty organizing tasks and activities

(6) Avoids, dislikes, or is reluctant to engage in tasks that require sustained mental effort

(7) Loses things necessary for tasks or activities (e.g., school assignments, pencils, books)

(8) Is easily distracted by extraneous stimuli

(9) Is forgetful in daily activities

(10) Fidgets with hands or feet or squirms in seat

(11) Leaves seat in classroom or in other situations in which remaining seated is expected

(12) Runs about or climbs excessively in situations in which remaining seated is expected

(13) Has difficulty playing or engaging in leisure activities quietly

(14) Is "on the go" or often acts as if "driven by a motor"

(15) Talks excessively

(16) Blurts out answers before questions have been completed

(17) Has difficulty waiting in line

(18) Interrupts or intrudes on others (butts into conversations or games)

(19) Loses temper

(20) Actively defies or refuses to comply with adult's requests or rules

(21) Is angry or resentful

(22) Is spiteful and vindictive

(23) Bullies, threatens, or intimidates others

(24) Initiates physical fights

(25) Lies to obtain goods for favors or to avoid obligations ("cons" others)

(26) Is physically cruel to people

(27) Has stolen items of nontrivial value

(28) Deliberately destroys others' property

(29) Is fearful, anxious, or worried

(30) Is self-conscious and easily embarrassed

(31) Is afraid to try new things for fear of making mistakes

(32) Feels worthless or inferior

(33) Blames self for problems; feels guilty

(34) Feels lonely, unwanted, or unloved; complains that "no one loves him or her"

(35) Is sad, unhappy, or depressed

| Symptoms | Points |
|---|---|
| Never | 0 |
| Occasionally | 1 |
| Often | 2 |
| Very often | 3 |

## Academic performance

(1) Reading

(2) Mathematics

(3) Written expression

## Classroom behavioral performance

(4) Relationship with peers

(5) Following directions

(6) Disrupting classes

(7) Assignment completion

(8) Organizational skills

| Performance Responses | Points |
|---|---|
| Excellent | 1 |
| Above average | 2 |
| Average | 3 |
| Somewhat of a problem | 4 |
| Problematic | 5 |

## Tallies

(1) Total questions answered 2 or 3 in symptom questions 1 to 9

(2) Total questions answered 2 or 3 in symptom questions 10 to 18

(3) Total questions answered 2 or 3 in symptom questions 19 to 28

(4) Total questions answered 2 or 3 in symptom questions 29 to 35

(5) Total questions answered 4 or 5 in performance questions 1 to 8

Total symptom score for questions 1 to 18 = SUM (points for symptoms questions 1 to 18); average performance score = SUM (points for all 8 performance questions) / 8

| Diagnosis | Symptom Questions | Performance Questions |
|---|---|---|
| Predominantly inattentive subtype ADHD | Score >= 2 in 6 of 9 from questions 1 to 9 | Score 4 or 5 on >= 1 |
| Predominantly hyperactive impulsive ADHD | Score >= 2 in 6 of 9 from questions 10 to 18 | Score 4 or 5 on >= 1 |
| ADHD-Combined inattention hyperactivity | Score >= 2 in 6 of 9 from questions 1 to 9 AND 6 of 9 from questions 10 to 18 | Score 4 or 5 on >= 1 |
| Oppositional defiant/ conduct disorder screen | Score >= 2 in 3 of 10 from questions 19 to 28 | Score 4 or 5 on >= 1 |
| Anxiety/depression screen | Score >= 2 in 3 of 7 from questions 29 to 35 | Score 4 or 5 on >= 1 |

**Source:** The National Initiative for Children's Healthcare Quality (NICHQ) Vanderbilt Assessment Scales. Available at www.nichq.org/resoures/toolkit and www.utmen.edu/pediatrics/general/clinical/behavior/aap_ADHD_toolkit/.

# Conners' Rating Scales-Revised (CRS-R)
## (C. K. Conners)

*Conners' Rating Scales-Revised (CRS-R)* is an instrument that uses observer ratings and self-report ratings to help assess ADHD and evaluate problem behavior in children and adolescents. The CRS-R instruments are used for routine screenings in schools, mental health clinics, residential treatment centers, pediatric offices, juvenile detention facilities, child protective agencies, and outpatient settings.

## Instrument(s) Description

Conners' Parent Rating Scales Revised
*Long Version (CPRS-R: L)*
The CPRS-R: L contains 80 items. It is typically used with parents or caregivers when comprehensive information and DSM-IV consideration are required.

## Scales include

- Oppositional
- Cognitive problems/inattention
- Hyperactivity
- Anxious-shy
- Perfectionism
- Social problems
- Psychosomatic
- Conners' Global Index
- DSM-IV Symptom Subscales
- ADHD Index

The CPRS-R: L also includes a Treatment Progress ColorPlot™ Form for proper age and gender profiling of scale scores.

**Short Version (CPRS-R: S)**:  The CPRS-R: S contains 27 items and covers a subset of the subscales and items on the long parent form. Scales include:

- Oppositional
- Cognitive problems/inattention
- Hyperactivity
- ADHD Index

---

## Sample Items

The CPRS provides a series of statements that the parent responds to regarding the child's behavior for the past month. The response is in a Likert type format, using the following categories:

- Not true at all (Never, Seldom)
- Just a little true (Occasionally)
- Pretty much true (Often, Quite a bit)
- Very much true (Very often, Very frequent)

## The first six items for the CPRS

1. Angry and resentful
2. Difficulty doing or completing homework
3. Is always "on the go" or acts as if driven by a motor
4. Timid, easily frightened
5. Everything must be just so
6. Has no friends

## Validity/Norms

Norms were based on a sample of 8000+ children and adolescents, males and females ages 3 to 17. Minority group samples were represented. Standardized data were based on the means and standard deviations for groups of children with ADHD and children without psychological problems.

## Administer to

*For the CRS-R:* parents and teachers of children and adolescents ages 3-17 and adolescent self-report ages 12-17.
*For the CAARS:* age 18 and older.

## Ordering Information

These forms can be ordered from Pearson Assessments at: www.pearsonassessments.com.

# Conners-Wells' Adolescent Self-Report Scale (CASS)
## (C. K. Conners and K.C. Wells)

**Long Form (CASS: L)**

The CASS: L contains 87 items and is appropriate for adolescents between the ages of 12 and 17. Typically used with adolescents when extensive information and DSM-IV consideration are required. Scales include:

- Family problems
- Emotional problems
- Conduct problems
- Cognitive problems/inattention
- Anger control problems
- Hyperactivity
- ADHD Index
- DSM-IV Symptom Subscales

The CASS: L also includes a Treatment Progress ColorPlot Form for proper age and gender profiling of scale scores.

**Short Form (CASS: S)**

The CASS: S contains 27 items and is designed for adolescents between the ages of 12 and 17. Scales include:

- Conduct problems
- Cognitive problems/inattention
- Hyperactivity
- ADHD Index

**Ordering Information**

These forms can be ordered from Pearson Assessments at: www.pearsonassessments.com.

# Conners' ADHD DSM-IV Scales (CADS)
## (C. K. Conners)

## Parent (CADS-P)

The CADS-P contains 26 items and features the option of having parents complete both or just 1 of the 2 subcomponents. The 26-item form includes the ADHD Index items and DSM-IV Symptom Subscale. The form allows the clinician to indicate whether the respondent should complete 1 or both subscales.

## Teacher (CADS-T)

The QuikScore form for this scale has been constructed like the CADS-P to allow for the optional administration of the subcomponents. Although this scale contains 27 items, teachers can complete just 12 items or just 18 items.

## Adolescent (CADS-A)

This scale consists of 30 items and elicits meaningful results whether just a subcomponent or the entire scale is administered.

Subscales for CADS-P, CADS-T, CADS-A:

- ADHD Index (12 items)
- DSM-IV Symptom Subscales (18 items)
- DSM-IV Inattentive (9 items)
- DSM-IV Hyperactive-Impulse (9 items)

## Ordering Information

These forms can be ordered from Pearson Assessments at: www.pearsonassessments.com.

# Information for Parents about
# Attention-Deficit/Hyperactivity Disorder (ADHD)

## What Is ADHD

ADHD is the name of a group of behaviors found in many children and adults. People with ADHD have trouble paying attention in school, at home, or at work. They may be much more active and/or impulsive than what is usual for their age. These behaviors contribute to significant problems in relationships, learning, and behavior. For this reason, children with ADHD are sometimes seen as being "difficult" or as having behavior problems. ADHD is common, affecting 4 to 12% of school-age children. It is more common in boys than in girls.

## What Are the Symptoms of ADHD

The child with ADHD who is inattentive will have 6 or more of the following symptoms:
- Difficulty following instructions
- Difficulty keeping attention on work or play activities at school and at home
- Loses things needed for activities at school and at home
- Appears not to listen
- Doesn't pay close attention to details
- Seems disorganized
- Has trouble with tasks that require planning ahead
- Forgets things
- Is easily distracted

The child with ADHD who is hyperactive/impulsive will have at least 6 symptoms:
- Runs or climbs inappropriately
- Is fidgety
- Can't play quietly
- Blurts out answers
- Interrupts people
- Can't stay in seat
- Talks too much
- Is always on the go
- Has trouble waiting his or her turn

## What Causes ADHD

Children with ADHD do not make enough chemicals in key areas in the brain that are responsible for organizing thought. Without enough of these chemicals, the organizing centers of the brain don't work well. This causes the symptoms in children with ADHD. Often there is a family history of ADHD. Things that don't cause ADHD: poor parenting (although a disorganized home life and school environment can make symptoms worse); too much or too little sugar, Aspartame, food additives or colorings; lack of vitamins; food allergies or other allergies; fluorescent lights; video games; or too much TV.

## What Can I Do to Help My Child With ADHD

A team effort, with parents, teachers, and doctors working together, is the best way to help your child. Children with ADHD tend to need more structure and clearer expectations. Families may benefit from talking with a specialist in managing ADHD-related behavior and learning problems. Medicine also helps many children. Talk with your doctor or nurse practitioner about treatments he/she recommends.

## What Medicines Are Used to Treat ADHD

Some of the medicines for ADHD are methylphenidate, dextroamphetamine, and bupropion. These medicines improve attention/concentration and decrease impulsive and overactive behaviors.

## What Can I Do at Home to Help My Child

Children with ADHD may be difficult to parent. They may have trouble understanding directions. Children with ADHD are often in a constant state of activity. This can be challenging. You may need to change your home life a bit to help your child. Here are some things you can do to help:

- Make a schedule. Set specific times for waking up, eating, playing, doing homework, doing chores, watching TV or playing video games, and going to bed. Post the schedule where your child will always see it. Explain any changes to the routine in advance.

- Make simple house rules. It's important to explain what will happen when the rules are obeyed and when they are broken.

- Make sure your directions are understood. Get your child's attention and look directly into his or her eyes. Then tell your child in a clear, calm voice specifically what you want. Keep directions simple and short. Ask your child to repeat the directions back to you.

- Reward good behavior. Congratulate your child when he/she completes each step of a task.

- Make sure your child is well supervised. Because they are impulsive, children with ADHD may need more adult supervision than other children their age.

- Watch your child around his or her friends. It's sometimes hard for children with ADHD to learn social skills. Reward good play behaviors.

- Set a homework routine. Pick a regular place for homework, away from distractions such as other people, TV and video games. Break homework time into small parts and allocate frequent breaks.

- Focus on effort, not grades. Reward your child when he or she tries to finish schoolwork, not just for good grades. You can give extra rewards for earning better grades.

- Talk with your child's teachers. Find out how your child is doing at school--in class, at playtime, at lunchtime. Ask for daily or weekly progress notes from the teacher.

# Information for Teens and Children
# About Attention-Deficit/Hyperactivity Disorder (ADHD)

"You're not paying attention." "Don't you know where you put your lunch money?" "Stop fidgeting!" "Don't interrupt."  Can you imagine what it would be like to hear people talk to you this way every single day? If you can imagine it, or if it sounds just like what you're used to hearing, then you know what it's like to have attention-deficit/hyperactivity disorder, or ADHD for short.

Kids who have ADHD are not "bad," "lazy," or "stupid." They have a behavior disorder, which means they may have problems paying attention or have trouble sitting still in their seats. They can also act on impulse -- this means doing things without thinking about them first. Kids with ADHD may spend a lot of time in the principal's office. They also might change their friends a lot.

## Who Gets ADHD

On average, 5 out of 100 kids have ADHD. That means that if your school has 500 kids, 25 may have ADHD -- that's like one whole class! Kids who have ADHD usually start having problems before they are 7 years old. Sometimes the problems begin when they start going to school. Boys have ADHD more often than girls, but no one knows why.

In fact, no one is sure why anyone has ADHD, although scientists and doctors think that it probably has to do with different levels of brain activity. No one gets ADHD on purpose, so it isn't ever anyone's fault. And ADHD isn't contagious -- you can't catch it from someone like the flu. A kid might have a bigger chance of developing ADHD if one of his relatives already has ADHD.

## What is ADHD

ADHD stands for attention-deficit/hyperactivity disorder. ADHD is a disorder that affects the brain. It causes people to behave differently from others. People with ADHD have problems in 1 or 2 major ways. The first is that they may have trouble focusing on tasks or subjects. The second is that they may act on impulse (without thinking), which can lead to negative consequences. That's why ADHD gets a bad rap.

### Symptoms and Signs of ADHD

The first type of ADHD includes problems with paying attention, staying organized, remembering things, problems completing work at school or home, difficulty following instructions, losing or forgetting things (e.g., homework). This type used to be called attention-deficit disorder, or ADD.

The second type involves hyperactivity and impulsivity and includes fidgeting, feelings of restlessness, difficulty awaiting your turn, and interrupting others.

The third type, which is the most common, involves a combination of the other two types.  If you have ADHD, you may not be aware that you are behaving in a way that's different from others; you're just doing what comes naturally. But you might notice that it's hard for you to pay attention. You might feel bored or frustrated in class. You may have a hard time getting started on assignments and finishing your work. Homework may take you much longer to complete.

ADHD can affect social situations, too. For example, you might react to someone by just saying what's on your mind -- what comes naturally -- and then you may get the feeling that you've shocked or offended the person or don't understand why people get mad at you. Some of the symptoms of ADHD can be difficult to deal with and can make a teen experience many different emotions. The more you understand about ADHD, the more involved you can be in your own treatment.

## What Medicines are Used to Treat ADHD

Some medicines used to treat ADHD are called psychostimulants. They can help people with ADHD to focus their attention better on things.

## School Tips for Helping Yourself with ADHD

If you have a study hall available to you during one class period or after school, use it and take advantage of a quiet time to study and complete homework.

Take notes during class. This can help to keep you focused on the material being taught.
Use your assignment book to keep lists of things to do. Don't make lists on scraps of paper -- you may end up losing them or forgetting about them. Get into the habit of completing a list of things to do each evening for what you want to accomplish the next day.

Talk to your teachers about your ADHD and how it affects your work. Ask for their assistance in areas you are experiencing problems. They will be more willing to help if they understand that you are trying to overcome these problems rather than making excuses. Sit in front of the classroom. This will help you to focus on the lesson and will enable you to pay attention and will minimize distractions.

Be prepared. If you are constantly going to class unprepared, buy a box of pens and keep them in your locker. Buy several small pocket-size notebooks. Each morning, if you find you don't have a pen and paper, use a small pocket-size notebook, and take a pen from your locker.

If you end up each day at home without the books needed to complete your assignments, use different methods to remember which books to bring home. Ask the school about bringing home an extra set of books. You will not need to carry your books back and forth and will never forget your books at home or school.

Find a partner to help you. Find someone you trust and work well with to help you stay focused during the day. Have a special signal they can give you if they see you have lost your focus.
Clean out your locker every Friday. Get into the habit of bringing home all loose papers in your locker each Friday. When you get home, you can sort through to see what you need and organize the papers. Having a clean locker will help you to stay organized and be prepared.
Believe in yourself and your abilities. You can succeed in what you do.

Check out this helpful Web site for children, teens and adults with ADHD: National Resource Center for ADHD, available at www.chadd.org.

# Internet Resources

### American Academy of Child and Adolescent Psychiatry
www.aacap.org
This Web site is an excellent source of information on the assessment and treatment of child and adolescent mental health disorders. Handouts for use with families (i.e., *Facts for Families*) are available on a multitude of problems, including ADHD.

### American Academy of Pediatrics (AAP)
www.aap.org
This Web site has excellent information for healthcare providers and parents on a variety of mental health topics, including ADHD. The AAP worked with the National Initiative for Children's Healthcare Quality to develop an evidence-based ADHD toolkit to assist practitioners in providing comprehensive care for children with this disorder.

### Children and Adults with Attention-Deficit/Hyperactivity Disorder (CHADD)
www.chadd.org
This national nonprofit organization was founded in 1987 in response to the frustration and sense of isolation experienced by parents and their children with ADHD.

### National Initiative for Children's Healthy Quality (NICHQ)
www.nichq.org/resources/toolkit
The NICHQ worked with experts to identify and categorize resources to assist clinicians to care for children with ADHQ. The ADHD toolkit can be downloaded at this Web site.

### National Institute of Mental Health
www.nimh.gov
This outstanding Web site has multiple educational handouts on a variety of mental health disorders, including ADHD, and links to informative Web sites.

### National Resource Center on ADHD:
http://www.help4ADHD.org/
This resource center is a program of CHADD, funded through a cooperative agreement with the Centers for Disease Control and Prevention.

# References

Magyary, D., & Brandt P (2002). A decision tree and clinical paths for the assessment and management of children with ADHD. *Issues Mental Health Nursing*, 23(6): 553-566.

Olson, B.G., Rosenbaum P.F., Dosa N.P., et al (2005). Improving guideline adherence for the diagnosis of ADHD in an ambulatory pediatric setting [In Process Citation] *Ambul Pediatr*, 5(3): 138-142.

Valente, S.M. (2001). Treating attention deficit hyperactivity disorder. *Nurse Practitioner*, 26(9): 14-15, 19-20, 23-27; quiz 27-29.

# Information for Healthcare Providers about Overweight/Obesity

## Quick Facts

- Calculation of body mass index (BMI) percentile is vital to identify children (3 years of age or older) who are overweight/obese.

- Currently, it is estimated that 20-30% of all children are overweight (greater than the 95th BMI percentile) or at risk for overweight.

- The number of overweight/obese children has more than tripled in the last 2 decades.

- Children and teens who are overweight/obese are at risk for hypertension, dyslipidemia, type 2 diabetes, polycystic ovary disease, worsened reactive airways disease, obstructive sleep apnea, metabolic syndrome, increased incidence of musculoskeletal complaints, gastroesophageal reflux, cardiovascular disease, nonalcoholic steatohepatitis, and poor coping outcomes.

- Parents and clinicians often fail to recognize child overweight/obesity.

- Overweight adolescents have a 70% chance of becoming overweight/obese adults, a risk that increases to 80% if 1 parent is overweight or obese.

- Children 3 to 6 years of age whose BMI is greater than the 85th percentile have a greater than 40% chance of being obese at age 25.

- Restrictive dieting and/or singling out 1 child in a family for weight loss is not effective and in fact more often leads to a greater likelihood of weight gain and/or the development of eating disorders (i.e., bulimia, binge eating).

## Critical History-Taking Questions

- Thorough assessment of eating patterns
- Thorough assessment of activity patterns
- Thorough assessment of mental health status and possible co-morbid mental health conditions
- Thorough assessment of symptoms related to possible co-morbid physiological conditions

## Medical Conditions That Should be Ruled Out

- Hypertension
- Dyslipidemia
- Type 2 diabetes
- Cushing's disease
- Obstructive sleep apnea
- Worsened asthma
- Insulin resistance
- Polycystic ovary syndrome
- Hypothyroidism
- Nonalcoholic steatohepatitis
- Gastroesophageal reflux
- Genetic syndromes (i.e., Prader Willi, Turner's syndrome, Laurence-Moon-Bardet-Biedl syndrome)
- Concomitant mental health problems
  - Depression
  - Anxiety
  - Eating disorder (e.g., bulimia, compulsive/binge eating)

## Blood Work/Tests That Might Be Helpful

- All overweight/obese children or teens should have the following testing: a fasting glucose, hemoglobin A1c, fasting lipid panel, liver function tests, free T4 and TSH.

- Other tests to be considered, given historical information, include: amylase/lipase levels, prolactin level, ultrasound of ovaries and/or liver, LH/FSH ratio, upper GI, pulmonary function tests, electrolytes with erythrocyte sedimentation rate and complete blood count, and possibly a sleep study.

## Medications and Drugs That May Add to Overweight in Children

- Steroids
- Antidepressants
- Mood stabilizers (e.g., lithium, valproate)
- Other psychotropic drugs (e.g., *Zyprexa, Risperdal*)
- Contraceptives (e.g., *Depo Provera*)

## Evidence-Based Interventions for Overweight/Obesity in Children and Teens

Interventions should focus on health, not weight.

There is some evidence to support that the most effective interventions for overweight/obese children are multifaceted (i.e., they target nutrition, exercise, and cognitive-behavior skills building) and are delivered in the context of the family.

# Information for Healthcare Providers about Eating Disorders

## Quick Facts

- Currently, more than 10 million people are afflicted with eating disorders and, of those, 87% are children and teens under the age of 20 years.

- Approximately 7% of adolescent males and 13% of adolescent females struggle with eating disorders.

- Eating disorders tend to occur in early to mid-adolescence, ranging from 13 years to 18 years of age; however, they are now occurring in younger children. Overindulgent eating patterns emerge earlier as well.

- Correlates of eating disorders include overweight status, low self-esteem, depression, anxiety, suicidal ideation, obsessive-compulsive traits, and substance use.

## Disordered Eating Patterns Include

- Anorexia nervosa
- Bulimia nervosa
- Binge/compulsive eating disorder
- Eating disorder not specified
- Antecedents of bulimia nervosa and anorexia nervosa include perfectionism and negative self-evaluation.

## Bulimia Nervosa has Been Found to be Influenced by

- Parental obesity
- Childhood obesity
- Critical comments by family about body shape, weight, or eating
- Early menarche
- Parental psychiatric disorder
- Certain parental problems (e.g., low contact and high expectations, and alcohol use)

## A Thorough Mental Health Evaluation is Necessary

Teens with eating disorders often have co-morbid mental health disorders (e.g., anxiety, depression) that also must be ruled out.

## The Following Laboratory Tests Should Be Considered

- Serum electrolytes
- Renal function tests
- Complete blood count
- Liver function tests
- Electrocardiogram

# DSM-IV Criteria for the Diagnosis of Eating Disorders

## Anorexia Nervosa

## DIAGNOSTIC FEATURES

The essential features of anorexia nervosa include refusal to maintain a minimally normal body weight, intense fear of gaining weight, and significant disturbance in the perception of the shape or size of one's body. In addition, postmenarcheal females with this disorder are amenorrheic. (The term anorexia is a misnomer because loss of appetite is rare.)

### Diagnostic Criteria for Anorexia Nervosa

| |
|---|
| A. Refusal to maintain body weight at or above a minimally normal weight for age and height (e.g., weight loss leading to maintenance of body weight less than 85% of expected; or failure to make expected weight gain during period of growth, leading to body weight less than 85% of that expected) |
| B. Intense fear of gaining weight or becoming fat, even though underweight |
| C. Disturbance in the way in which one's body weight or shape is experienced, undue influence of body weight or shape on self-evaluation, or denial of the seriousness of the current low body weight |
| D. In postmenarcheal females, amenorrhea (i.e., the absence of at least 3 consecutive menstrual cycles) |

**Specify type:** *Restricting Type:* During the current episode of anorexia nervosa, the person has not regularly engaged in binge-eating or purging behavior (i.e., self-induced vomiting or the misuse of laxatives, diuretics, or enemas).

*Binge-Eating/Purging Type:* During the current episode of anorexia nervosa, the person has regularly engaged in binge-eating or purging behavior (i.e., self-induced vomiting or the misuse of laxatives, diuretics, or enemas).

**PREVALENCE** Rates of 0.5 to 1% among females in late adolescence and early adulthood.

**COURSE** The mean age of onset for anorexia nervosa is 17 years, with some suggesting bimodal peaks at ages 14 and 18 years. The onset is often associated with a stressful life event, such as leaving home for college. The course and outcome are highly variable. Some individuals recover fully after a single episode, while others relapse and experience a chronic debilitating course of the illness over many years.

# DSM-IV Criteria for the Diagnosis of Eating Disorders

## Bulimia Nervosa

## DIAGNOSTIC FEATURES

The essential features of bulimia nervosa are binge-eating and inappropriate compensatory methods to prevent weight gain. In addition, the self-evaluation of individuals with bulimia nervosa is excessively influenced by body shape and weight.

### Diagnostic Criteria for Bulimia Nervosa

| A. Recurrent episodes of binge-eating. An episode of binge-eating is characterized by both of the following:<br>(1) Eating, in a discrete period of time (e.g., within any 2-hour period), an amount of food that is definitely larger than most people would eat during a similar period of time and under similar circumstances<br>(2) A sense of lack of control over eating during the episode (e.g., a feeling that one cannot stop eating or control what or how much one is eating) |
| --- |
| B. Recurrent inappropriate compensatory behavior in order to prevent weight gain, such as self-induced vomiting; misuse of laxatives, diuretics, enemas, or other medications; fasting; or excessive exercise. |
| C. The binge-eating and inappropriate compensatory behaviors both occur, on average, at least twice a week for 3 months. |
| D. Self-evaluation is unduly influenced by body shape and weight. |
| E. The disturbance does not occur exclusively during episodes of anorexia nervosa. |

*Specify type: Purging Type:* During the current episode of bulimia nervosa, the person has regularly engaged in self-induced vomiting or the misuse of laxatives, diuretics, or enemas.

*Nonpurging Type:* During the current episode of bulimia nervosa, the person has used other inappropriate compensatory behaviors, such as fasting or excessive exercise, but has not regularly engaged in self-induced vomiting or the misuse of laxative, diuretics, or enemas.

**PREVALENCE** Approximately 1 to 3% among adolescent and young adult females. Approximately 1 male for every 10 females suffers from bulimia nervosa.

**COURSE** Bulimia nervosa usually begins in late adolescence or early adult life. The binge-eating frequently begins during or after an episode of dieting. Disturbed eating behavior persists for at least several years in a high percentage of clinic samples. The long-term outcome is not known.

*Reprinted with permission and adapted from the Diagnostic and Statistical Manual of Mental Disorders, Fourth Edition, Text Revision, Copyright 2000. American Psychiatric Association.*

# Screening Questions for Eating Disorders

## Questions for Parents

Are you concerned about your child's weight?

Does your son or daughter make negative comments about his or her weight?

## Questions for Children and Teens

Are you concerned about your weight?

Do you eat breakfast every day?

## Guidelines for Adolescent Preventative Services (GAPS) (AMA, 1994) (see Section One).

## Questions for the Younger Adolescent

Do you spend a lot of time thinking about ways to be skinny?

Do you do things to lose weight (e.g., skip meals, take pills, starve yourself, and vomit)?

Do you work, play, or exercise to make you sweat or breathe hard at least 3 times a week?

## Questions for the Middle to Older Adolescent

Are you satisfied with your eating habits?

Do you ever eat in secret?

Do you spend a lot of time thinking about ways to be thin?

In the past year, have you tried to lose weight or control your weight by vomiting, taking diet pills or laxatives, or starving yourself?

Do you exercise or participate in sports activities that make you sweat and breathe hard for 20 minutes or more at a time at least 3 times during the week?

# Information about Obesity/Overweight in Children and Teens for Parents

## What Is Considered Overweight or at Risk for Overweight in Children and Teens

Overweight in children is determined by their body mass index (BMI) percentile, not their BMI as in adults. Children found to be greater than the 85th percentile are considered to be at risk for overweight; however, children found to be greater than the 95th BMI percentile are considered to be overweight. These guidelines were established by many professional organizations including the American Academy of Pediatrics. If you are unsure whether your child or teen is overweight, have your child's healthcare provider calculate his or her BMI percentile for you or consult one of the many Web sites that will help you to calculate it.

## How Can Overweight Affect Someone's Health

Excessive weight can cause a wide variety of health problems, including:

- Type 2 diabetes
- High blood pressure
- Worsening of asthma
- Heart disease
- Sleep apnea
- Gastro-esophageal reflux
- Poor coping outcomes (e.g., depression, low self-esteem)

## What Causes Overweight

The point at which a person's nutritional intake exceeds his or her activity level causes an energy imbalance. If this energy imbalance is maintained over a long period of time, a person will store the extra energy as fat and put on extra weight.

## Which Children/Teens Are at Risk to Become Overweight

Scientists who study overweight in children and teens have identified factors that place certain children and teens at high risk for overweight.

Those risk factors include:

- Overweight in the toddler and preschool years
- Sedentary lifestyle (e.g., a lot of computer or television viewing time)
- Natural parents or caretakers who are overweight or have a complication of overweight/obesity
- Dietary intake of fatty foods and/or decreased intake of fruits and vegetables

## What Are the Treatments for Overweight in Children and Teens

It is important that overweight in children and teens be treated using the following 3 approaches, which focus on healthy lifestyle patterns:

- Healthy dietary intake
- Regular exercise or activity
- Positive emphasis on supportive and healthy lifestyles

## What Can You Do to Help Your Child with His or Her Weight

There are a few simple guidelines that you can initiate with your child or teen to help him or her to make positive, healthy lifestyle changes:

- Decrease the amount of sugared beverages that your child drinks (e.g., soda, fruit punch, and sports drinks).
- Decrease the amount of television viewing time and/or computer time to 1-2 hours per day.
- Provide a moderately low fat diet.
- Provide healthy snacks for your family.
- Engage in healthy family activities on a regular basis.
- Do not restrict your child's dietary intake only, rather change the whole family's diet to a healthy one.
- Be a positive and supportive influence on your child/teen and model regular healthy eating and activity habits.

# Information about Anorexia Nervosa
## in Children and Teens for Parents

## What Is Anorexia Nervosa

Anorexia nervosa is the most common eating disorder among girls entering puberty, although there is an increasing trend of adolescent boys developing this disorder. Anorexia nervosa is a disorder that makes eating very distressing. People who struggle with this disorder become very anxious or obsessed with maintaining or reducing their body weight through rigid control of their caloric intake. These people have intense fear of gaining weight and feel that their self-worth is directly affected by their body shape.

## What Are Common Signs and Symptoms of Anorexia Nervosa

- Weight loss
- Dietary restriction
- Food rituals
- Avoiding public eating
- Frequent weighing
- Excessive focus on exercise or dieting
- Loss of menstrual periods
- Hair loss or growth of baby-fine hair on face or body
- Feeling cold much of the time

## How Can Anorexia Nervosa Affect Someone's Health

It can cause:
- Low blood pressure
- Low heart rate
- An inability to concentrate
- Fatigue/muscle weakness
- Irritability
- Constipation
- Loss of menstrual periods/sterility
- Dehydration
- Brittle bones
- Kidney damage

## What Causes Anorexia Nervosa

There is much uncertainty about the causes of eating disorders. Although many people believe that both anorexia and bulimia can develop from a strict diet, the reasons that "a diet" turns into an eating disorder go beyond the desire to be thin and lose weight. For those teens with anorexia nervosa, the desire to be thinner and to restrict their eating habits is constantly on their mind. Anorexia literally means to lose one's appetite; however, people with anorexia nervosa do not truly lose their appetite. Instead, the fear of weight gain causes them to go on strict diets that may result in the inability to eat normally. People who struggle with anorexia nervosa feel driven to lose weight, and their desire to control their weight is tied to their self-worth. They often feel that eating is a sign of a lack of self-control.

Some people who develop anorexia nervosa may have emotional needs that are not being met in their lives. They may have difficulty in social relationships or have problems making friends. The development of anorexia nervosa is sometimes a physical way for adolescents to deal with overwhelming and emotional issues that can occur during the transition to adulthood. Still others develop anorexia nervosa in the face of puberty and the start of sexual feelings. This may be related to concerns about their own sexuality, normal body changes that occur with puberty, or an unpleasant sexual experience.

It is very common for teens with anorexia nervosa to be high achievers and perfectionists; however, they feel that they are underachievers. Frequently, teens with anorexia nervosa set high standards for themselves that are often impossible to achieve. As a result, they are left with feelings of failure and inadequacy.

## What Are the Treatments for Anorexia Nervosa

Treatment for anorexia nervosa involves the professional help of a trained psychiatrist or other mental health provider who specializes in eating disorders. Medications, such as antidepressants or anti-anxiety medications are used along with intensive counseling. Nutritional counseling by a trained specialist is often included. Anorexic teens who have fasted for long periods often will not be able to eat normal amounts of food and will need to begin eating small amounts of food more often. The digestive tract of someone who has dieted extremely may have difficulty digesting certain foods until their system becomes used to eating more food. Some anorexics need to be admitted to the hospital if their weight loss is so extreme that the person's health is poor (e.g., if their heart rate or blood pressure becomes too low).

## What Can You Do If You Think Your Child Has Anorexia Nervosa

If you believe that your child may have anorexia nervosa, you should seek professional help from his or her doctor or nurse practitioner right away. The longer that your child has fixed patterns and attitudes toward eating, the more difficult it will be to begin to change those habits. It may feel very upsetting and scary for your child to think of changing these habits.

Specialists will be able to offer you many suggestions, even if your child is uncertain that he or she would like to change things. Below are some suggestions that other people have said have been helpful to them. Help your child to:

- Find ways to pamper him or herself that have nothing to do with food (perhaps something that he or she used to enjoy).
- Put his or her energy into different channels. Find activities that your child is good at or that give him or her satisfaction.
- Try to do what he or she wants to do, not just what other people want him or her to do, at least some of the time.
- Focus on finding ways to like him or herself that do not involve a "target weight" or anything to do with eating.
- Believe that he or she can overcome this problem and get the help needed to do it NOW!

# Important Information about Bulimia Nervosa in Children and Teens for Parents

## What Is Bulimia Nervosa

Bulimia nervosa is an eating disorder that commonly occurs in adolescent girls and rarely occurs in males. It is defined by episodes of "binge" eating or eating large quantities of food in a short time. This behavior may be severe with very large quantities of food being eaten, often containing carbohydrates. People who struggle with bulimia try to prevent weight gain that would normally occur after bingeing by following the binge-eating with periods of food restriction, vomiting, laxative abuse, and/or excessive exercising (otherwise known as "purging"). In severe cases, when vomiting is used, the binge episodes may become more common with the cycles repeating over several hours. Without treatment, the severity of this eating disorder increases and the teen's life becomes more chaotic and focused on purging behavior. The drive to eat is so strong that the teen may steal food in order to satisfy his or her compulsion. Teens with this disorder are usually ashamed of their behavior, so they often keep their bingeing secret.

## Who Has Bulimia Nervosa

Many people don't know when a family member or friend has bulimia because the binge-eating and purging (ridding the body of calories by laxative use, vomiting, or excessive exercise) occurs in private and there may not be noticeable weight loss or weight gain.

## What Are Common Signs or Symptoms of Bulimia Nervosa

- Dental cavities
- Enlarged parotid glands, which are by the back portion of the face below the jaws
- Puffy cheeks
- Uncontrollable gastro-esophageal reflux
- Abdominal pain and bloating
- Constipation
- Secret eating or large amounts of food disappearing
- Excessive exercise
- Preoccupation with food
- Going to the bathroom directly following meals
- Using laxatives and vomiting to control weight
- Intestinal problems from frequent laxative use
- Kidney problems from use of "water" pills (diuretics)
- Irregular heartbeat
- Muscle weakness or fatigue

## What Causes Bulimia Nervosa

Eating disorders are caused by a variety of factors, some that we know about and some that we do not. Worry or stress may be one cause, especially worry about getting fat. Dieting and missing meals as a form of weight control may trigger food cravings and overeating. Sometimes bulimia can develop as a complication of some emotional trauma or upsetting event, such as family breakdown, death of a friend or relative, or abuse. Other risk factors for the development of bulimia include poor self-esteem, extreme anxiety, and a highly sensitive nature.

## What Are the Treatments for Bulimia Nervosa

Counseling by a trained psychiatrist or mental health provider/counselor is one of the primary treatments used for people with this disorder. This therapy should help the person to understand the complex emotions that trigger bingeing and purging behaviors. The counseling is often directed toward the person's distorted self-image, uncontrollable and excessive eating, profound guilt, and embarrassment. Treatment usually includes the use of antidepressants and/or other medications to help the obsessive thinking and uncontrollable compulsive behaviors. Occasionally, some teens need to be admitted to the hospital if their fluid loss is extreme and/or health is threatened (e.g., if heart rate becomes too irregular or if blood pressure becomes too low).

## What Can I Do to Help

- Strongly suggest that the teen get help
- Be positive and supportive
- Be empathetic to the teen's feelings
- Go to a support group
- Don't blame the teen
- Give written information that encourages the teen to get help early

# Information about Bulimia Nervosa for Teens

## What Is Bulimia Nervosa

Bulimia nervosa is an eating disorder that most commonly occurs in adolescent girls and rarely occurs in males. It is defined by episodes of "binge" eating or eating large quantities of food in a short time. This behavior may be severe with very large amounts of food being consumed, often containing carbohydrates. Teens who struggle with bulimia try to prevent weight gain that would normally occur after binge-eating by not eating for a period of time, vomiting, laxative abuse and/or excessive exercising (otherwise know as "purging"). In severe cases when vomiting is used, the bingeing may become more frequent. Without treatment, this disorder can become severe. The drive to eat can become so strong that people with this disorder may even steal food to satisfy their compulsive eating. Teens are often ashamed of their behavior, so they often binge in secret.

## Who Has Bulimia Nervosa

Many people don't know when a family member or friend has bulimia because the binge-eating and purging (ridding the body of calories by laxative use, vomiting, or excessive exercise) often occurs in private, and there may not be visible weight loss or weight gain.

## What Are Common Signs or Symptoms of Bulimia Nervosa

- Dental cavities
- Enlarged parotid glands, which are in the back portion of the face, below the jaws
- Puffy cheeks
- Uncontrollable stomach acid that comes up in the throat
- Abdominal pain and bloating
- Constipation
- Secret eating or large amounts of food disappearing
- Excessive exercise
- Preoccupation with food
- Going to the bathroom directly following meals
- Using laxatives and vomiting to control weight
- Intestinal problems from frequent laxative use
- Kidney problems from use of "water" pills (diuretics)
- Irregular heartbeat
- Muscle weakness or fatigue

## What Causes Bulimia Nervosa

Eating disorders are caused by many things, some that we know about and some that we do not. Worry or stress may be one cause, especially worry about getting fat. Dieting and missing meals as a form of weight control may trigger food cravings and overeating. Sometimes bulimia can develop after an emotional trauma or upsetting event (e.g., family breakdown, death of a friend or relative, abuse). Other risk factors for the development of bulimia include poor self-esteem, extreme anxiety, and a highly sensitive nature.

## What Are the Treatments for Bulimia Nervosa

Counseling by a trained psychiatrist or mental health provider/counselor is one of the primary treatments used for teens with this disorder. This therapy helps teens to understand the complex emotions that trigger these bingeing and purging behaviors. Counseling is often directed toward the teen's distorted self-image as well as the excessive eating and guilt. Treatment often includes the use of antidepressants and/or other medications to help the obsessive thinking and compulsive behaviors. Some teens need to be admitted to the hospital if their fluid loss is extreme and/or their health is threatened (e.g., if their heart rate becomes too irregular or if their blood pressure becomes too low).

## What Can I Do

If you think that you or a friend has this eating disorder, talk to your doctor/nurse practitioner, parent, or trusted adult about it right away. The earlier that treatment is started, the better. You won't be helping yourself or your friend by keeping it a secret.

# Internet Resources

### American Academy of Child and Adolescent Psychiatry
www.aacap.org
This Web site is an excellent source of information on the assessment and treatment of child and adolescent mental health disorders. Handouts for use with families (i.e., *Facts for Families*) are available on a multitude of problems, including eating disorders.

### American Academy of Pediatrics
www.aap.org
This Web site contains information for both healthcare providers and parents, including excellent clinical practice guidelines and handouts.

### Bright Futures in Practice: for Nutrition, Physical Activity, and Mental Health
www.brightfutures.org
This Web site contains outstanding materials for health professionals on a variety of topics that can be easily implemented in practice.

### Centers for Disease Control and Prevention
www.cdc.gov
The CDC Web site contains outstanding materials for healthcare professionals and the public on a variety of topics, including the latest information on overweight and obesity.

### National Association of Pediatric Nurse Practitioners' KySS Program
www.napnap.org
This website contains information about the KySS Program and its initiatives and materials.

### National Eating Disorders Association
www.nationaleatingdisorders.org/
The National Eating Disorders Association (NEDA) is the largest not-for-profit organization in the United States that works to prevent eating disorders and provide treatment referrals to those suffering from anorexia, bulimia, and binge-eating disorder and to those concerned with body image and weight issues. NEDA is dedicated to expanding public understanding of eating disorders and promoting access to quality treatment for those affected along with support for their families through education, advocacy, and research. The organization develops prevention programs for a wide range of audiences, publishes and distributes educational materials, and operates the nation's first toll-free eating disorders information and referral helpline.

# References

American Psychiatric Association (2000). *Diagnostic and Statistical Manual of Mental Disorders, Fourth Edition* (DSM-IV). Washington, DC: APA.

Kaye, D.L., Montgomery, M.E., & Munson, S. (2002). *Child and Adolescent Mental Health.* Philadelphia, PA: Lippincott.

Jellinek, M., Patel, B.P., & Froehle, M. (2002). *Bright Futures in Practice: Mental Health- Vol I. Practice Guide.* Arlington, VA: National Center for Education in Maternal        and Child Health.

Jellinek, M., Patel, B.P., & Froehle, M. (2002). *Bright Futures in Practice: Mental Health- Vol II. Tool Kit.* Arlington, VA: National Center for Education in Maternal and Child Health.

Melnyk, B.M., Brown, H., Jones, D.C., Kreipe, R., & Novak, J. (2003). Improving the mental/psychosocial health of U.S. children and adolescents. Outcomes and implementation strategies from the national KySS summit. *Journal of Pediatric Healthcare*, 17 (6: Supplement 1): S1- S24.

## Information for Healthcare Providers about
## Helping Children Cope with Grief and Loss

### What Is Grief

Grief is the term used for the many feelings and behaviors we experience and manifest when we are faced with loss. The loss may be from the death of a significant other, relocation, or divorce. Grief is a natural and normal reaction to loss and change. Children **do** experience grief as they have feelings and are aware of losses. However, children grieve differently based upon their development and personality.

### Difference between Grief and Mourning

Grief can be thought of as the internal experience related to a loss. Mourning and bereavement are terms used interchangeably and are the outward manifestations of grief.

The goal of working with children who are grieving is to assist them in externalizing their internal experience

### Feelings Children May Experience While Grieving

| | | |
|---|---|---|
| Abandonment | Confusion | Guilt |
| Anger | Denial | Panic |
| Anxiety | Depression | Rejection |
| Body Distress | Fear | Sadness |

Children may experience one or more of these feelings. It is important to give children a vocabulary to help them **identify**, **label**, and **express** these different feelings.

## Children's Developmental Perceptions of Death

Children's developmental level and understanding of death will have an impact on their experience of grief.

**Ages 0-2 years:** Children react the way they see their caretakers react. They may resist change and separation from caretakers.

**Ages 3-5 years:** Children do not accept death as permanent. They will often inquire when the deceased person will return. They react primarily to separation.

**Ages 5-9 years:** Children accept permanency but not universality at this age. Questions about why their loved one had to die and not someone else are a central theme.

**Ages 9-12 years:** Children see death as permanent and universal. They take death personally and understand they will also die someday. They are interested in concrete details about the death, funeral, burial, etc.

**Age 12 years and older:** Adolescents have reached an adult understanding of death. They spend significant time thinking about death and trying to understand what happens after death. They have very intense emotions during this time.

## Behavioral Reactions in Children Experiencing Grief

Children will normally act out some of their feelings. In a supportive way, let children know what behavior you see that has changed. Continue to expect that the child will function. It is important to set limits on aggressive behavior and respond to regressive behavior. As the child heals, the regressive behavior should dissipate.

| | |
|---|---|
| Adult role behaviors | Temper outbursts |
| Disinterest in usual activities | Panic attacks |
| Headaches | Regression |
| Increased dependency on adults | Silence |
| Model child behaviors | Stomachaches |
| Over-activity | Withdrawal |

## Four Tasks of Childhood Grieving

Children and adults grieve differently. Adults often feel sad over an extended period of time, whereas children's grief is more intermittent. Children's expression of grief may erupt and then be over relatively quickly as they move on to the next activity. It will then erupt again at another time, only to go away again. This "volcano"-like mourning, though different from that experienced by adults and possibly uncomfortable for adults, is a normal grief pattern for children.

Nussbaum (1998) identified four tasks that assist children and adolescents in adjusting to the death. These tasks are not linear; each child will go through these tasks in his or her own way and time. Activities to assist children with these tasks are included in the parent handouts. The tasks are:

1. Understanding: acknowledging the reality of death
2. Identifying and expressing feelings
3. Commemorating/honoring the person who died
4. Going on - not "getting over"

As children progress through the different developmental stages, they **re-grieve** the loss and seek to understand their loss in new ways. This can be confusing and difficult for the adults in the children's lives. Adults need to understand this to assist in improving the emotional health of their children.

## Differential Symptoms of Depression and Grief

The symptoms of depression and grief are similar. Table 6.1 highlights some of the differences between the two. If a parent has any concerns about how a child is progressing through grief or whether a child has slipped into depression, it is best to contact a counselor familiar with children and grief. The local hospice or the counselors at the child's school are potential resources.

## Table 6.1 Symptoms of Depression and Grief

| Depression | Grief |
|---|---|
| 1. Missed school or poor school performance | 1. Missed school or poor school performance |
| 2. Changes in eating and sleeping habits | 2. Changes in eating and sleeping habits |
| 3. Withdrawal from friends and activities once enjoyed | 3. Withdrawal from friends and activities once enjoyed |
| 4. Persistent sadness and hopelessness | 4. Intense and intermittent sadness and hopelessness |
| 5. Indecision, forgetfulness and lack of concentration | 5. Indecision, forgetfulness, and lack of concentration |
| 6. Poor self-esteem or feelings of guilt | 6. Feeling different from other children or feeling guilty |
| 7. Overreaction to criticism | 7. Overreaction to criticism |
| 8. Frequent physical complaints, such as headaches and stomachaches | 8. Frequent physical complaints, such as headaches and stomachaches |
| 9. Anger and rage | 9. Anger and rage |
| 10. Lack of enthusiasm, low energy or motivation | 10. Either low energy or extra-high energy (may appear like ADHD), low motivation to perform well |
| 11. Drug/alcohol abuse | 11. Drug/alcohol abuse |
| 12. Thoughts of death or suicide or thoughts about wanting to die | 12. Thoughts about death and dying |

*Adapted from: National Mental Health Association. Child and adolescent depression. Available at.http://www.nmha.org/children/green1/child_depression.cfm.*

## Complicated Grief

Grief may be complicated by death that involves trauma, homicide, suicide, multiple losses, or a significant change in function. Children with complicated grief may have more of the many feelings previously mentioned, and these feelings will be more intense. Anger, resentment, and confusion are common. These children need more assistance with expression, and it is best to seek help from a children's counselor or mental health professional. Children who experience trauma and grief are at risk for posttraumatic stress disorder.

# How Parents Can Help Children/Teens
# to Cope With Loss and Grief

## What Is Grief
Grief is the term used for the many feelings and behaviors we experience when we are faced with loss. The loss may be from the death of a significant other, relocation, or divorce. Grief is a normal reaction to loss and change. Children **do** experience grief as they have feelings and are aware of losses. However, children grieve differently based upon age and personality.

## What Are Some of the Feelings Children May Have
Children may have one or more of these feelings: abandonment or the feeling of being left alone, anxiety, confusion, anger, guilt, fear, body distress, rejection, sadness, and panic. It is important to help children identify, label, and talk about these different feelings.

## What Is the Effect of Age on Children Who Are Grieving
Children's development and age will have an impact on how they think about death and the loss.

| Age | Reaction |
| --- | --- |
| **Infants and young children (0 - 2 years)** | React the way they see their caretakers react. They may resist change and separation from caretakers. |
| **Preschool aged children (3 - 5 years)** | Do not accept death as permanent. They will often ask when the deceased person will return. They may react primarily to separation. |
| **Young school-aged children (5 - 9 years)** | Accept that death is permanent, but not universal. Questions about why their loved one had to die and not someone else are common. |
| **Older school-aged children (9 -12 years)** | See death as permanent and universal. They take death personally and understand they also will die someday. They are interested in concrete details about the death, such as the funeral and burial. |
| **Older children (12 years and older)** | Have started to reach an adult understanding of death. They spend a significant amount of time thinking about death and trying to understand what happens after death. They have very intense emotions during this time. |

As children go through the different developmental stages, they re-grieve the loss and try to understand their loss in new ways. This can be confusing and difficult for adults.

## What Are Some of the Behaviors You May See in Your Child Who Is Grieving

Children will normally act out some of their feelings. In a supportive way, let children know what behavior you see that has changed. Continue to expect that the child will function. It is important to set limits on destructive behavior and to respond to a less mature or regressive behavior. As the child heals, the regressive behavior should disappear.

Temper outbursts, panic attacks, regression or less mature behavior, disinterest in usual activities, increased dependency on adults, stomachaches and headaches, silence, model child behaviors or trying to be "the perfect child," withdrawal, adult role behaviors or taking on adult responsibilities, over-activity.

## What Is the Difference Between Grief and Mourning

Grief can be thought of as the internal experience about a loss. Mourning and bereavement are words that people use about the outward signs of grief. The goal of dealing with children who are grieving is to help them to talk about how they feel.

## What Is the Difference Between Grief and Depression

The symptoms of depression and grief are similar. If you have any concerns about how your child is adjusting to the loss or whether a child has slipped into depression… TALK TO SOMEONE! People that can help you are nurses, doctors, nurse practitioners, school counselors, and psychologists.

## How do Children Grieve Differently than Adults

Adults often feel sad over an extended period of time, whereas children's grief tends to come and go. Children's expression of grief may flare up and then be over relatively quickly as they move on to the next activity. This "volcano"-like mourning, though different from that experienced by adults and possibly uncomfortable for adults, is a normal grief pattern for children.

# How Can I Help My Child Deal With Loss and Grief?

The following tasks help the child in adjusting to a loss. Each child will complete these tasks in his or her own way and on his/her own time schedule. The below suggestions may help you.

| Task | Activities to Assist Child |
|---|---|
| **Understanding: facing the reality of death** | • Offer the child time to talk about death and loss as he/she experiences it in everyday life. Allow the child to tell his or her "story" of the death of the loved one.<br>• Be there to listen, including long after you think the child should be moving on, as he or she will revisit this grief throughout his/her life.<br>• Answer questions about death and loss as honestly as possible. |
| **Identifying and expressing feelings** | • Show the child how you talk about feelings and help the child identify and express feelings.<br>• Tell the child that his/her feelings are normal and that others feel the same way.<br>• Offer age-appropriate expressions of feelings such as: writing about feelings; talking to someone about feelings; crying; laughing; snuggling; singing; arts and crafts; walking or other physical activity like dance and martial arts.<br>• Read age-appropriate books with the child and discuss his/her understanding of the story. |
| **Commemorating/ honoring the person who died** | • Assist your child with creating an ongoing list and put it on the refrigerator: "Things I remember about _____" and have family members contribute to it when they want.<br>• Help your child write a story, poem, prayer, or song for the loved one.<br>• Assist your child in creating a memory book or box with photographs and/or items.<br>• Take your child to the cemetery. Take flowers or a balloon.<br>• Plant a tree or some flowers with your child in honor of the loved one. |
| **Going on - not "getting over"** | • Create a ritual to say good-bye to the loved one.<br>• Ask your child to create a collage of the things that make him/her happy to be alive.<br>• Express and validate the child's mixed feelings about "going on."<br>• Develop rituals around anniversary dates for remembering the loved one. |

*Adapted from: Nussbaum, K. (1998). Preparing the Children: Information and Ideas for Families Facing Terminal Illness and Death. Burnsville, North Carolina: Compassion Books.*

# Information for Teens about Coping with Loss and Grief

## What Is Grief

Grief is the term used for the many feelings and behaviors we experience when we are faced with loss. The loss may be from the death of a significant other, relocation, or divorce. Grief is a natural and normal reaction to loss and change. Teens do experience grief as they have feelings and are aware of losses. However, everyone experiences grief differently.

## What Are Some of the Feelings I May Have

You may have 1 or more of these feelings: abandonment or the feeling of being left alone, anxiety, confusion, anger, guilt, fear, body distress, rejection, sadness, and panic. It is important to try to identify, name, and talk about these different feelings with your parent, a health professional, or counselor.

## Some Teens Who Are Grieving May Notice Some of These Behaviors

Temper outbursts, panic attacks, regression or less mature behavior, disinterest in usual activities, increased dependency on adults, stomachaches and headaches, silence, or trying to be "the perfect child," withdrawal, taking on adult activities, over-activity. If you notice any of these changes in your behavior, again, share this with your parent, a health professional, or counselor.

## What Is the Difference between Grief and Depression

The symptoms of depression and grief are similar. If you have any concerns about how you are adjusting to your loss or wondering if you are depressed.......TALK TO SOMEONE! People that can help you are nurses, doctors, nurse practitioners, school counselors, and psychologists.

## How do Teens Grieve Differently than Adults

Adults often feel sad over an extended period of time, whereas a teen's grief tends to come and go. Your expression of grief may flare up and then be over quickly as you move on to the next activity. This "rollercoaster" feeling, though different from that experienced by adults and possibly uncomfortable for adults, is a normal grief pattern for teens.

# What Can I Do to Help Myself Deal with Loss and Grief?

There are certain tasks that help people adjust to a loss. Every person will complete these tasks in his or her **own** time and in his/her own way. The below suggestions may help you.

## Understanding: facing the reality of death

1. Take the time to talk about death and loss as you experience it in everyday life. Tell your "story" of the death of your loved one.
2. Find someone who will listen -- a parent, a trusted adult, a health professional, or counselor.
3. Find someone who will listen long after you think you should be moving on, as you will revisit this grief in some way throughout your life.
4. Ask questions about death and loss.

## Identifying and expressing feelings

1. Notice how other people talk about feelings.
2. Try to identify and express your feelings.
3. Try one of these activities:
   - ♥ writing about feelings
   - ♥ talking to someone about feelings
   - ♥ snuggling
   - ♥ art and crafts
   - ♥ physical activity like dance, martial arts.
   - ♥ crying
   - ♥ laughing
   - ♥ singing
   - ♥ walking

## Commemorating/honoring the person who died

1. Create an ongoing list and put it on the refrigerator: "Things I remember about _____" and have family members contribute to it when they want.
2. Write a story, poem, prayer, or song for the loved one.
3. Create a memory book or box with photographs and/or items.
4. Plan a visit to the cemetery with your family. Take flowers or a balloon.
5. Plant a tree or some flowers in honor of the loved one.

## Going on - not "getting over"

1. Create a ritual to say good-bye to the loved one.
2. Create a collage of the things that make you happy to be alive.
3. Express your mixed feelings about "going on."
4. Develop rituals around anniversary dates for remembering the loved one.

*Adapted from: Nussbaum, K. (1998). Preparing the Children: Information and Ideas for Families Facing Terminal Illness and Death. Burnsville, North Carolina: Compassion Books.*

# Internet Resources

## Compassion Books
www.compassionbooks.com

This Web site describes many books and resources available for professionals, families, and children related to loss and grief. Materials available on the Web site are reviewed by professionals who are current in experience, practice, and research.

## The Dougy Center for Grieving Children & Families
www.dougy.org/

This site has educational information for professionals, parents, and children about grief. There are also many excellent links to other resources and training materials to help you work with grieving children.

# References

Fox, S. (1988). *Good Grief: Helping Groups of Children When a Friend Dies.* Boston, MA: New England Association for the Education of Young Children.

Harting, L. B., Tompkins, J.M., & Ryan-Weneger, N.A. (2004). Grief masks. *Journal of Pediatric Healthcare*, 18: 308-309.

National Mental Health Association. Child and adolescent depression. Available at: http://www.nmha.org/children/green1/child_depression.cfm.

Nussbaum, K. (1998). *Preparing the Children: Information and Ideas for Families Facing Terminal Illness and Death.* Burnsville, NC: Compassion Books.

# Information for Healthcare Providers about
# Mood Disorders; Management and Medications

## Quick Facts

- Mood disorders are common, affecting about 5% of children (males and females equally) and 10 to 20% of teens (females twice as often as males).
- The mean age of onset for a major mood disorder is 14 years, and 8 years for dysthymia.
- Reoccurrence of a mood disorder is as high as 50 to 70%.
- The risk in children/teens is increased if 1 or more parents is depressed.
- An estimated 40 to 70% of affected children/teens have mental health comorbidities (e.g., anxiety disorders; substance use, conduct disorders, ADHD).
- Depression is a risk factor for other high-risk behaviors and often precedes substance abuse by about 4 years.

## Common Presenting Complaints

- Irritability, anger, behavior problems, sleep problems, decline in school performance, lack of interest in usual activities, and somatic complaints (e.g., stomachaches, headaches).
- Younger children (younger than 9 years of age) who are depressed can present with restlessness/irritability and can be misdiagnosed with ADHD.

## Risk Factors for Depression

- Parental depression or other family mental health problems
- Family dysfunction, including domestic violence and marital conflict
- Societal or family violence or abuse, physical or sexual abuse
- Acute or chronic illness
- Life stressors and changes, trauma and/or losses
- Poor self-esteem and poor coping skills
- Attachment issues and lack of social or peer support, social isolation
- Substance abuse or other psychopathology

## Mood Disorders are a Major Risk Factor for Suicide

- Suicide is the third leading cause of death in teens (5 to 10% of high school students make attempts every year).
- Suicidality increases with age.
- The age group with the highest incidence of suicide is older male teens.
- Girls make more attempts at suicide, but males are more successful.

## Predictors/Major Risk Factors for Suicide

- Degree of hopelessness (This is the #1 predictor of suicide.)
- Family history of suicide or recent suicide in school
- Method available (e.g., gun, medications)
- Prior history of self-harming behaviors or impulsivity
- Depression and/or a sudden change in mood
- Drug and alcohol abuse
- Inability to "contract for safety"
- Serious medical illness
- Family violence

## Assessment of Depression

## Consider

- Onset and development of symptoms; context in which symptoms occur/are sustained
- Biological/psychosocial stressors
- Comorbid psychopathology
- Impact of symptoms on activities of daily living and family
- Parent-child interactions
- Developmental history
- Coping behaviors and styles, sleep, and rhythmicity

## Medical History

- Medical visits/hospitalizations (e.g., recurrent pain syndromes)
- Medical disorders (e.g., hypothyroidism, anemia, chronic illness) and medications

## School History

- Academic, athletic, social, and behavioral functioning
- Potential versus actual achievements
- Pattern of attendance and school nurse visits

## Social History

- Environmental stressors, separations, and losses
- Involvement with peers/withdrawal, giving away prized possessions

## Family History

- Family mental health history (e.g., anxiety/mood disorders)
- Family medical history (e.g., headaches, chronic illness, recurrent pain)
- Parental responses to medications [e.g., Selective Serotonin Reuptake Inhibitors (SSRIs)]

## Interview with the Child/Adolescent

## Consider

- The child's/adolescent's report of symptoms and sense of functional impairment
- Objective signs of depression (e.g., loss/gain of weight, hypo/hyperactivity)
- Depending on development, engage the child in play, drawing, or other artistic expression. Also, obtain history from collateral contacts.

## Diagnoses That Should Be Ruled Out With Depression if Suspected From History

- Hypothyroidism (obtain TSH, FT4)
- Anemia (obtain CBC with differential)
- Mononucleosis or chronic fatigue syndrome (obtain monospot)
- Eating disorders
- Substance use or withdrawal -- e.g., alcohol, cocaine, amphetamines, opiates (obtain toxicology screen)
- Premenstrual syndrome
- Diabetes (obtain fasting serum glucose)
- Head trauma or CNS lesions
- Cushing syndrome
- HIV/AIDS
- Mitral valve prolapse
- Systemic lupus erythematosus
- Developmental delay
- Failure to thrive
- Seizures
- Lead intoxication (obtain lead level)
- Medication side effects -- e.g., benzodiazepines, beta-blockers, clonidine, corticosteroids, *Accutane*, oral contraceptives

## Assess for Suicidal Ideation/Intent, Plan, and Means

If depression is suspected or patients make self-harming comments, **ALWAYS** ask about:
- Suicidal ideation
- Plan and means
- Intent
- **Suicide warning signs:** change in behavior (giving away treasured items), mood (sudden upswing in mood), thinking (preoccupation with death), major life changes (major illness or death of a loved one)

## Management of Suicidal Ideation

- Option if low-risk for suicide: Contract for safety and mobilize social supports (A safety contract is included in this guide).
- Options if high-risk for suicide: Call 911; transport to ED
- In-home crisis intervention programs
- Depending on severity, consider: outpatient counseling, inpatient hospitalization or residential programs

## Management of Depression

- Assess for suicidal ideation. Teach about suicide warning signs and contract for safety. Caution families to remove drugs, alcohol, and weapons from the home.
- Educate the family about the depressive condition and support the child and family.
- The American Academy of Child and Adolescent Psychiatry recommends psychotherapy as the first treatment approach for depressed youth with mild to moderate depression.
- Involve school and after-care personnel; interdisciplinary collaboration is important.
- Careful and regular follow-up with the family is crucial.
- Medications should be reserved for severe depression and should be prescribed in conjunction with counseling therapy.
- SSRIs (*Celexa, Paxil, Zoloft, Prozac, Effexor*) are the recommended first-line treatment. It is extremely important to start antidepressant medication at <u>LOW</u> doses in children and adolescents and increase dosage <u>SLOWLY</u>. A trial of 8 weeks is recommended; it usually takes 4-6 weeks to see an effect. Antidepressants should be used for 6 to 9 months, weaned slowly, and never stopped abruptly. Avoid tricyclic antidepressants in patients with suicidal ideation due to the potential for cardiac toxicity with overdose.

*Note:* Caution must be exercised when prescribing SSRIs to children and adolescents with psychiatric disorders, ( see table 7.1) as studies have shown an increased risk of suicidal thinking and behavior (suicidality) in the first few months of starting treatment. Patients started on SSRIs should be observed closely for worsening of symptoms, suicidality, or unusual changes in behavior. Families should be advised to monitor for these signs/symptoms and alert the provider if they are present.

**\*Table 7.1 Prescribing Selective Serotonin Reuptake Inhibitors**

| SSRIs (recommended order of preference) | Usual Starting Dose (SD) and Effective Daily Dosage (DD) | | Common Side Effects | Important Considerations |
|---|---|---|---|---|
| - Fluoxetine | (SD): | 5 mg | Fairly common: | Monitor weekly somatic symptoms, heart rate, and blood pressure. Assess therapeutic levels when initiating and increasing dosage. |
| (*Prozac*) | (DD): | 10-20 mg | Excitation Agitation | |
| -Citalopram (*Celexa*) | (SD): (DD): | 5 mg 10-20mg | Nausea Vomiting Diarrhea | *Celexa* and *Zoloft* are the least activating; *Prozac* is very stimulating in children/teens. |
| - Sertraline (*Zoloft*) | (SD): (DD): | 12.5-25 mg 50-100 mg | Dizziness Chills | *Prozac* has a long half life (13-15 days), which may potentate interactions with another drug if introduced too early after discontinuation. |
| - Paroxetine (*Paxil*) | (SD): (DD): | 5-10 mg 20-40 mg | Less common: Muscle twitching | |
| - Fluvoxamine (*Luvox*) | (SD): (DD): | 25 mg 50-200 mg | Fever Confusion Diaphoresis Suicidal ideation | *Paxil* currently carries a caution about increasing suicidal ideation. |
| *Prozac* is the only FDA-approved medication for child/teen depression. | | | Rare: Seizures Delirium Coma | |

\* WARNING: SSRIs MAY INCREASE SUICIDAL IDEATION IN CHILDREN AND ADOLESCENTS.

Updated and adapted from: Melnyk, B.M. & Moldenhauer, Z.M. (1999). Current approaches to the assessment, management, and prevention of child and adolescent depression. *Advance for Nurse Practitioners 7(2): 24-29, 97.*

# DSM-IV Criteria for Dysthymic Disorder

## Diagnostic Features

Dysthymic disorder is a chronically depressed mood that occurs for most of the day more days than not for at least 2 years. Individuals with dysthymic disorder describe their mood as sad or "down in the dumps." In children, the mood may be irritable rather than depressed, and the required minimum **duration is only 1 year**.

## Diagnostic Criteria for Dysthymic Disorder

| |
|---|
| A.  Depressed mood for most of the day, for more days than not, as indicated either by subjective account or observation by others, for at least 2 years.<br><br>*Note:* In children and adolescents, mood can be irritable and duration must be at least 1 year. |
| B. Presence, while depressed, of 2 (or more) of the following:<br><br>    (1) Poor appetite or overeating<br><br>    (2) Insomnia or hypersomnia<br><br>    (3) Low energy or fatigue<br><br>    (4) Low self-esteem<br><br>    (5) Poor concentration or difficulty making decisions<br><br>    (6) Feelings of helplessness |
| C. During the 2-year period (1 year for children or adolescents) of the disturbance, the person has never been without the symptoms in criteria A and B for more than 2 months at a time. |
| D. No depressive episode has been present during the first 2 years of the disturbance (1 year for children and adolescents). |
| E. There has never been a manic episode, a mixed episode, or a hypomanic episode, and criteria have never been met for cyclothymic disorder. |
| F. The disturbance does not occur exclusively during the course of a chronic psychotic disorder, such as schizophrenia or delusional disorder. |
| G. The symptoms are not due to the direct physiological effects of a substance (e.g., a drug of abuse, a medication) or a general medical condition (e.g., hypothyroidism). |

H. The symptoms cause clinically significant distress or impairment in social, occupational, or other important areas of functioning.

*Specify if:* ***Early Onset:*** if onset is before 21 years of age

*Late onset:* if onset is age 21 years or older

## PREVALENCE

The prevalence of dysthymic disorder has been estimated at approximately 3%.

## COURSE

Dysthymic disorder often has an early and insidious onset (i.e., in childhood, adolescence, or early adult life) as well as a chronic course. In clinical settings, individuals with dysthymic disorder usually have superimposed major depressive disorder, which is often the reason for seeking treatment. If dysthymic disorder precedes the onset of major depressive disorder, there is less likelihood that there will be spontaneous full interepisode recovery between major depressive episodes and a greater likelihood of having more frequent subsequent episodes.

# DSM-IV Criteria for Major Depressive Episode

## DIAGNOSTIC FEATURES

The essential feature of a major depressive episode is a period of at least 2 weeks during which there is either depressed mood or the loss of interest or pleasure in nearly all activities. In children and adolescents, the mood may be irritable rather than sad.

## Criteria for Major Depressive Episode

A. Five (or more) of the following symptoms have been present during the same 2-week period and represent a change from previous functioning; at least 1 of the symptoms is either (1) depressed mood or (2) loss of interest or pleasure.

(1) Depressed mood most of the day, nearly every day, as indicated by either subjective report (e.g., feels sad or empty) or observation made by others (e.g., appears tearful). Note: In children and adolescents, can be irritable mood.
(2) Markedly diminished interest or pleasure in all, or almost all, activities most of the day, nearly every day (as indicated by either subjective account or observation made by others)
(3) Significant weight loss when not dieting or weight gain (e.g., a change of more than 5% of body weight in a month), or decrease or increase in appetite nearly every day. Note: In children, consider failure to make expected weight gain.
(4) Insomnia or hypersomnia nearly every day.
(5) Psychomotor agitation or retardation nearly every day (observable by others, not merely subjective feelings of restlessness or being slowed down)
(6) Fatigue or loss of energy nearly every day
(7) Feelings of worthlessness or excessive or inappropriate guilt (which may be delusional) nearly every day (not merely self-reproach or guilt about being sick)
(8) Diminished ability to think or concentrate, or indecisiveness, nearly every day (either by subjective account or as observed by others)
(9) Recurrent thoughts of death (not just fear of dying), recurrent suicidal ideation without a specific plan, or a suicide attempt or a specific plan for committing suicide.

B. The symptoms do not meet criteria for a mixed episode.

C. The symptoms cause clinically significant distress or impairment in social, occupational, or other important areas of functioning.

D. The symptoms are not due to the direct physiological effects of a substance (e.g., a drug of abuse, a medication) or a general medical condition (e.g., hypothyroidism).

E. The symptoms are not better accounted for by bereavement, i.e., after the loss of a loved one, the symptoms persist for longer than 2 months or are characterized by marked functional impairment, morbid preoccupation with worthlessness, suicidal ideation, psychotic symptoms, or psychomotor retardation.

## PREVALENCE

Major depression occurs in approximately 2% of children and up to 5% of adolescents.

## COURSE

Symptoms of a major depressive episode usually develop over days to weeks. A prodromal period that may include anxiety symptoms and mild depressive symptoms may last for weeks to months before the onset of a full major depressive episode. The duration of a major depressive episode is also variable. An untreated episode typically lasts 6 months or longer, regardless of age at onset.

*Reprinted with permission and adapted from the Diagnostic and Statistical Manual of Mental Disorders, Fourth Edition, Text Revision, Copyright 2000. American Psychiatric Association.*

# DSM-IV Criteria for Bipolar Disorder

## DIAGNOSTIC FEATURES

The essential feature of bipolar I disorder is a clinical course that is characterized by the occurrence of 1 or more manic episodes or mixed episodes. Often, individuals have also had 1 or more major depressive episodes. The essential feature of bipolar II disorder is a clinical course that is characterized by the occurrence of 1 or more major depressive episodes accompanied by the occurrence of at least 1 hypomanic episode.

### Diagnostic Criteria for a Manic Episode

| Elevated, expansive, or irritable mood lasting at least 1 week, accompanied by at least 3 of the following: |
| --- |
| • Inflated self-esteem or grandiosity |
| • Decreased need for sleep |
| • Flight of ideas or racing thoughts |
| • Distractibility |
| • Increase in goal-directed activity or psychomotor agitation |
| • Excessive involvement in pleasurable activities that have a high potential for negative consequences (e.g., buying sprees, sexual activity) |
| • Juveniles appear less likely to have distinct "episodes"; frequent (up to multiple times daily) episodes or mixed states are more commonly described in younger patients. |

## PREVALENCE

Bipolar disorder occurs in 1% of female and male adolescents.

## COURSE

Bipolar disorder is a recurrent disorder. More than 90% of individuals who have a single manic episode go on to have future episodes.

# Screening Tools for Depression

As with other mood disorders, depression should not be diagnosed solely by a screening tool. Further evaluation in the form of a clinical interview is necessary for children and adolescents identified as depressed through a screening process. Further evaluation also is warranted for children or adolescents who exhibit depressive symptoms but who do not screen positive.

There are a few valid and reliable depression screening tools for children and adolescents. In adults, the U.S. Preventive Task Force recommends asking the following 2 questions, which may be as effective as using longer screening instruments. These questions may be indicated when interviewing teens, especially if time is limited for the use of longer screening instruments.

1.  Over the past 2 weeks, have you ever felt down, depressed, or hopeless?

2.  Over the past 2 weeks, have you felt little interest or pleasure in doing things?

From: Agency for Healthcare Research and Quality, Rockville, Md. Screening for Depression. What's New from the USPSTF. AHRQ Publication No. APPIP02-0019, May 2002. Available at: http://www.ahrq.gov/clinic/3rduspstf/depression/depresswh.htm.

Section 7
Mood Disorders

# Center for Epidemiological Studies Depression Scale for Children (CES-DC)
## (L.S. Radloff)

## Description

The **Center** for **Epidemiological Studies** Depression Scale for Children (CES-DC) (see the instrument on the following page) is a 20-item self-report depression inventory with possible scores ranging from 0 to 60. Each response to an item is scored as follows:

0 = "Not At All"
1 = "A Little"
2 = "Some"
3 = "A Lot"

However, items 4, 8, 12, and 16 are phrased positively, and thus are scored in the opposite order:
3 = "Not At All"
2 = "A Little"
1 = "Some"
0 = "A Lot"

Higher CES-DC scores indicate increasing levels of depression. Weissman and colleagues (1980), the developers of the CES-DC, have used the cut-off score of 15 as being suggestive of depressive symptoms in children and adolescents. That is, scores over 15 can be indicative of significant levels of depressive symptoms.

## Psychometric Properties

The CES-DC has been found to be a valid and reliable tool for depression screening in older school-age children and adolescents.

## References

Faulstich, M.E., Carey, M.P., Ruggiero, L., et al. (1986). Assessment of depression in childhood and adolescence: an evaluation of the Center for Epidemiological Studies Depression Scale for Children (CES-DC). *American Journal of Psychiatry*, 143(8): 1024-7.

Weissman, M.M., Orvaschel, H., Padian, N. (1980) Children's symptom and social functioning self-report scales: comparison of mothers' and children's reports. *Journal of Nervous Mental Disorders*, 168(12):736-40.

*From: Bright Futures at Georgetown University, available at www.brightfutures.org; in the public domain.*

# BRIGHT FUTURES TOOL FOR PROFESSIONALS

## Center for Epidemiological Studies
## Depression Scale for Children (CES-DC)

Number _____

Score _____

## INSTRUCTIONS

Below is a list of the ways you might have felt or acted. Please check how much you have felt this way during the past week.

| DURING THE PAST WEEK | Not At All | A Little | Some | A Lot |
|---|---|---|---|---|
| 1. I was bothered by things that usually don't bother me. | ❏ | ❏ | ❏ | ❏ |
| 2. I did not feel like eating, I wasn't very hungry. | ❏ | ❏ | ❏ | ❏ |
| 3. I wasn't able to feel happy, even when my family or friends tried to help me feel better. | ❏ | ❏ | ❏ | ❏ |
| 4. I felt like I was just as good as other kids. | ❏ | ❏ | ❏ | ❏ |
| 5. I felt like I couldn't pay attention to what I was doing. | ❏ | ❏ | ❏ | ❏ |

| DURING THE PAST WEEK | Not At All | A Little | Some | A Lot |
|---|---|---|---|---|
| 6. I felt down and unhappy. | ❏ | ❏ | ❏ | ❏ |
| 7. I felt like I was too tired to do things. | ❏ | ❏ | ❏ | ❏ |
| 8. I felt like something good was going to happen. | ❏ | ❏ | ❏ | ❏ |
| 9. I felt like things I did before didn't work out right. | ❏ | ❏ | ❏ | ❏ |
| 10. I felt scared. | ❏ | ❏ | ❏ | ❏ |

| DURING THE PAST WEEK | Not At All | A Little | Some | A Lot |
|---|---|---|---|---|
| 11. I didn't sleep as well as I usually sleep. | ❏ | ❏ | ❏ | ❏ |
| 12. I was happy. | ❏ | ❏ | ❏ | ❏ |
| 13. I was more quiet than usual. | ❏ | ❏ | ❏ | ❏ |
| 14. I felt lonely, like I didn't have any friends. | ❏ | ❏ | ❏ | ❏ |
| 15. I felt like kids I know were not friendly or that they didn't want to be with me. | ❏ | ❏ | ❏ | ❏ |

| DURING THE PAST WEEK | Not At All | A Little | Some | A Lot |
|---|---|---|---|---|
| 16. I had a good time. | ❏ | ❏ | ❏ | ❏ |
| 17. I felt like crying. | ❏ | ❏ | ❏ | ❏ |
| 18. I felt sad. | ❏ | ❏ | ❏ | ❏ |
| 19. I felt people didn't like me. | ❏ | ❏ | ❏ | ❏ |
| 20. It was hard to get started doing things. | ❏ | ❏ | ❏ | ❏ |

*From: Bright Futures at Georgetown University, available at www.brightfutures.org; in the public domain.*

# The Children's Depression Inventory (CDI)
## (M. Kovacs)

## Description

This is a 27-item scale used to assess severity of depressive symptoms experienced in the prior 2 weeks, in persons aged 7 to 17 years. The 3 forced-choice response format indicates severity, from absence of symptom (score = 0) to definite symptom (score = 2) (e.g., "I am sad once in a while"; "I am sad many times"; "I am sad all the time"). The severity of depression symptoms is rated: less than 15 = nondepressed, 15 to 21 = mildly depressed, 22 to 26 = moderately depressed, over 27 = severely depressed.

## Psychometric Properties

**Reliability:** Internal consistency reliability has been found to be good, with coefficients ranging from 0.71 to 0.89 with various samples. Test-retest reliability correlations appear to be acceptable. It is, however, expected that the symptoms of depression would change over time, and regression to the mean is associated with repeated testing over time.

**Validity:** Numerous research studies have supported the CDI as assessing important constructs both for explanatory and predictive uses for characterizing symptoms of depression in children and adolescents. Studies of discriminant validity found significant differences of negative mood factor scores ($p < .05$) but no significant difference for total CDI scores among a sample of 134 children and adolescents with various depressive disorders. Some studies report the CDI to successfully distinguish normals from diagnostic categories, while other studies have been less favorable, and it is agreed that more research on the discriminant validity is needed for the CDI.

| | |
|---|---|
| *Item 2*<br>Nothing will ever work out for me<br>I am not sure if things will work out for me<br>Things will work out for me O.K. | *Item 5*<br>I am bad all the time<br>I am bad many times<br>I am bad once in a while |
| *Item 3*<br>I do most everything O.K.<br>I do most things wrong<br>I do every thing wrong | *Item 6*<br>I think about bad things happening to me once in a while<br>I worry that bad things will happen to me<br>I am sure that terrible things will happen to me |

## Ordering Information

The CDI is available from: http://www.pearsonassessments.com.

# Postpartum Depression Screening Scale (PDSS)
## (C. Tatano-Beck, R. K. Gable)

The Postpartum Depression Screening Scale (PDSS), assists clinicians in identifying mothers suffering from postpartum depression early and easily.

## Description

This 35-item, self-report instrument can be administered in just 5 to 10 minutes. Used as a brief screening device, it identifies women who are at high risk for postpartum depression, so that healthcare professionals can then refer them for definitive diagnosis and treatment. Written at a third-grade reading level, PDSS items are brief and easy to understand. Mothers respond using a 5-point scale ranging from "strongly disagree" to "strongly agree." The test yields an overall severity score falling into 1 of 3 ranges:

Normal adjustment
Significant symptoms of postpartum depression
Positive screen for major postpartum depression

In addition, the PDSS provides scores for 7 symptom areas:

- Sleeping/eating disturbances
- Anxiety/insecurity
- Emotional lability
- Mental confusion
- Loss of self
- Guilt/shame
- Suicidal thoughts

## Psychometric Properties

### Validity/Norms

An Inconsistent Responding Index is also included to measure response validity. Standardization is based on 2 samples: 525 new mothers of various ethnic backgrounds and 150 women recruited through childbirth classes and newspaper ads prior to giving birth. The first 7 items on the scale can function as a Short Form. Completed in just a minute or two, this Short Form provides only a total score, though a woman's response to item 7 can be used to gauge her level of suicidal thinking. Given the high incidence of postpartum depression, the current low rate of detection, and the potentially serious consequences, the PDSS is extremely useful in identifying women who need focused attention from mental health professionals.

## Administration

The PDSS can be used across various specialties, including obstetrics, pediatrics, psychiatry, psychology, and social work. It can be administered as early as 2 weeks after delivery. In addition to indicating which mothers need to be referred for a complete diagnostic work-up and treatment, the scale guides and informs treatment by means of the symptom profile it produces. And its brevity and economy make the PDSS ideal for monitoring treatment response.

## Ordering Information

The PDSS is copyrighted and must be purchased for use. It can be ordered from Western Psychological Services (WPS), 12031 Wilshire Boulevard, Los Angeles, CA 90025-1251, or accessed at: http://www.wpspublish.com. Available in English and Spanish.

# Information on Depression for Parents

## What Is Depression

Depression is an unhappy mood that affects daily functioning, including thoughts, feelings, behavior, and overall health. When depression is too severe or lasts too long, it can be considered an illness. Left untreated, depression can take the joy out of life and even take away the desire to live. Everyone experiences minor upsets, but this does not mean that everyone is depressed. To have true depression, the symptoms must be present for at least 2 weeks.

## How Common Is Depression

Depression in children and teens is far more common than most people realize and affects girls and boys equally. After puberty, girls are twice as likely as boys to be depressed. Ten out of 100 teens get seriously depressed each year, and many more have mild levels of sadness or the blues. About 1 in 10 children without known problems has suicidal thoughts.

## What Are the Signs of Depression

The most important signs to look for are feelings of hopelessness and sadness. While every child or teen is sad some of the time, no child should feel sad all of the time. If you notice that your child is unhappy and can't seem to have fun, think of this as a sign of depression. To be hopeless or without hope means to feel that nothing can go right, that nothing will change, and that no one can help.

Poor self-esteem is another important sign of depression. This is the teen's or child's attitude toward himself. If your child's self-esteem is poor, he or she may feel stupid, ugly, or worthless. Another sign is a change in school performance. If your child was a good student and now wants to stay home, or if his/her grades suddenly fall, he/she may be depressed. Other signs include sleep problems, appetite changes, irritability, crying, and aches and pains, such as headaches or stomachaches.

What would your child say if he or she is depressed? Don't expect your child to say much, because you can't count on him/her telling you how he/she feels. While your child may talk of being unhappy, he or she probably won't say, "I'm depressed" the way an adult will. So, you want to be aware of the signs.

## What If My Child Should Mention Suicide

Sometimes a child mentions that he or she does not want to live. If your child mentions suicide: Take it seriously. Talk to your child. Ask if he or she has made a plan for suicide. If so, it is more serious. If suicide is mentioned or if an attempt is made, seek professional help immediately. Do not assume your child is just looking for attention. Don't ever dare a youngster who mentions suicide to "go ahead." You may think it's a bluff, but he or she may take the dare.

## How Can a Parent Help

You can be very helpful to your depressed child. Some suggestions include: Be supportive -- listen to what your child has to say. Encourage him or her to keep talking. If your child can't talk well with you, perhaps he or she can speak with a sibling, aunt, friend, teacher, or healthcare provider. Encourage your child to describe or write down how he or she feels. Don't get angry if he/she describes unhappy feelings. If the problem is severe, worrisome, or lasts more than 2 weeks, get professional help.

## What Are the Causes of Depression in Children

There is no single answer to the cause of depression. It is probable that several factors combine to create the condition. The child's environment, especially if it is unhappy and stressful, is often a major cause. Depression also may be triggered by difficult situations, such as a death or divorce in the family or abuse. Another possible contributing factor is heredity. Studies show that depression frequently runs in families, so genetics may play a part in the depression of some children. Yet another reason is a lack of a certain chemical in the brain, called serotonin.

## What Are the Treatments for Depression

- Treatment is possible and helpful. The choice of treatment depends on the cause of the problem, the severity of the depression, and whether suicidal thoughts are present. Psychotherapy is the primary treatment. By meeting regularly with a therapist, your child can find out the causes of his/her depression, and then learn ways to help deal with it. It is usually good for the family to become involved in the treatment.
- Medication can be an effective part of treatment. Antidepressants have few side effects and are not habit-forming or addictive.
- Finally, parents should not feel guilty if their child is depressed. The important point is to realize that there is a problem and to get help for it. If you are concerned, be sure to talk to your child's healthcare provider. Remember, childhood and teen depression is treatable.

# What Can I Do to Prevent or Help My Child with Depression

- Stay involved in your child's life. Spend time with your child regularly, even if it's only a family dinner. Too often, parents respond to growing teenagers' wishes for independence by withdrawing from their teens' lives. The most important thing for parents to do is to be aware of and involved in their teen's life.
- Support positive relationships by encouraging your teen to get involved in school, clubs, or community events. Help your teen find interests and activities where he or she can connect with other teens. Also, know where your teen is and what he/she is doing when they go out.
- Talk to your teen, and listen when he/she talks to you! Parents should talk to their children as often as possible so teens can talk about their problems and worries. Ask your teen about school and friends. Listen to his/her troubles and help find solutions.
- Teach your child coping and problem-solving skills; it also is important for you to model positive ways of coping and dealing with stress.
- Know the warning signs of depression and be aware if your child shows any of these signs while talking to you, especially if he or she mentions suicide. Praise your teen's accomplishments rather than finding fault with things he/she does. Teens need to feel that their parents care about them and that what they are doing is recognized.
- It is mainly your job to make sure that your child receives the treatment he or she needs. Make sure that your teen takes his/her medication and goes to counseling. Be supportive.
- For more information about depression, contact the school counselor, psychologist, or social worker at your child's school, or contact your child's doctor or nurse practitioner.

# Information on Depression for Teens

## What Is Depression

Depression is a common and serious condition that can affect your thoughts, feelings, behavior, and overall health. Ten out of 100 teens get seriously depressed each year, and many more have mild levels of sadness or the blues.

## When You're Depressed, You Might Feel or Act in Some of These Ways

- You feel sad or cry a lot and it doesn't go away.
- You feel guilty easily; you feel like you are no good; you've lost your confidence.
- Life seems empty or like nothing good is ever going to happen again.
- You have a negative attitude a lot of the time, or it seems like you have no feelings.
- You don't feel like doing a lot of the things you used to enjoy -- like playing music, sports, being with friends, going out -- and you want to be left alone most of the time.
- It's hard to make up your mind. You forget lots of things, and it's hard to concentrate.
- You get angry often. Little things make you lose your temper; you overreact.
- Your sleep pattern changes; you start sleeping a lot more or you have trouble falling asleep at night. Or, you wake up really early most mornings and can't get back to sleep.
- Your eating habits change; you've lost your appetite or you eat a lot more.
- You feel restless and tired most of the time.
- You think about death, or feel like you're dying, or have thoughts about hurting yourself or committing suicide.

## Some teens who are depressed also can get "manic" at times. When you're manic, you may feel or act in some of these ways

- You feel high as a kite... like you're "on top of the world."
- You get unreal ideas about the great things you can do- things that you really can't do.
- Thoughts go racing through your head and you talk a lot.
- You're a nonstop party, constantly running around.
- You do too many wild or risky things: with regard to driving, spending money, sex, etc.
- You're so "up" that you don't need much sleep.
- You're rebellious or irritable and can't get along at home or school, or with your friends.

## If you think you're depressed... TALK TO SOMEONE!

If you have had some of these symptoms and they have lasted a couple of weeks or have caused a big change in your routine, you should talk to someone who can help, like a psychologist, nurse or doctor, or your school counselor!

## Treatment for Depression

Having depression doesn't mean that a person is weak, or a failure, or isn't really trying... it means they need TREATMENT. Most people with depression can be helped with counseling, and some are helped with counseling and medicine.

COUNSELING means talking about feelings with a special healthcare provider who can help you with the relationships, thoughts, or behaviors that are causing the depression. Don't wait; ask your parents or your school counselor for help today. MEDICINE is used to treat more serious depression. These medications are not "uppers" and are not addictive. When depression is so bad that you can't focus on anything else, when it interferes with your life, medication might be necessary along with counseling. But most often, counseling alone works. With treatment, most depressed people start to feel better in just a few weeks.

## What about Suicide

Most people who are depressed do not commit suicide. But, depression increases the risk for suicide or suicide attempts. It is NOT true that people who talk about suicide do not attempt it. Suicidal thoughts, remarks, or attempts are ALWAYS SERIOUS... if any of these happen to you or a friend, you must tell a responsible adult IMMEDIATELY.... It's better to be safe than sorry.

## Why Do People Get Depressed

Sometimes people get seriously depressed after something like a divorce in the family, major money problems, the death of someone they love, a messed-up home life, or breaking up with a boyfriend or girlfriend. Other times, depression just happens. Often, teens react to the pain of depression by getting into trouble: trouble with alcohol, drugs, or sex; trouble with school or bad grades; problems with family or friends. This is another reason why it's important to get treatment for depression before it leads to other trouble.

## Myths about Depression

- MYTH: It's normal for teens to be moody; Teens don't suffer from "real" depression.
  FACT: Depression is more than just being moody; and it affects people at any age.
- MYTH: Telling an adult that a friend might be depressed is betraying a trust. If someone wants help, he or she will get it.
  FACT: Depression, which saps energy and self-esteem, interferes with a person's ability or wish to get help. It is an act of true friendship to share your concerns with an adult who can help. No matter what you "promised" to keep secret, your friend's life is more important than a promise.
- MYTH: Talking about depression only makes it worse.
  FACT: Talking about your feelings to someone who can help, like a psychologist or nurse practitioner, is the first step toward beating depression. Talking to a close friend also can provide you with the support and encouragement you need to talk to your parents or school counselor about getting help for depression.

# CONTRACT FOR SELF SAFETY

I, _____, promise to keep myself safe. If I am thinking about hurting myself, I will tell my parent, another close adult, or my nurse practitioner or doctor.

_____     _____
Signature of Adolescent                           Signature of Provider or
                                                              Parent/Guardian

_____
Date

# CONTRACT FOR OTHERS' SAFETY

I, _____, promise to keep others around me safe from harm. If I am thinking about hurting anyone, I will tell my parent, another close adult, or my nurse practitioner or doctor.

_____  
Signature of Adolescent

_____  
Signature of Provider or Parent/Guardian

_____  
Date

# Internet Resources

### About Our Kids
www.aboutourkids.org/.
This Web site contains a wealth of resources for families about child and adolescent mental health and parenting. Resources include science-based articles, newsletters, and manuals; a guide to common mental health problems; lists of recommended books, Web sites and organizations; a glossary of medical terms explained in an easy-to-understand format; and an ask-the-expert service. About Our Kids is presented by the New York University School of Medicine Child Study Center.

### American Academy of Child and Adolescent Psychiatry (AACAP):
www.aacap.org
This Web site contains information about research, legislative activities, and meetings regarding child and adolescent mental health; policy statements; clinical practice guidelines; and a directory of child and adolescent psychiatrists. It also offers a set of FACT SHEETS for families in English, Spanish, and several other languages on a variety of topics that include ADHD, bullying, depression, and suicide.

### National Institute of Mental Health
www.nimh.gov
This outstanding Web site offers multiple educational handouts on a variety of mental health disorders, including mood disorders, and links to other informative Web sites.

### Youth Depression Treatment and Prevention Programs
http://www.kpchr.org/public/acwd/acwd.html.
The following downloadable evidenced-based cognitive-behavioral intervention programs for adolescents, developed by Lewinsohn, Clark, and colleagues are available free of charge. These programs were developed for use by mental health professionals with groups of adolescents who are depressed or at risk for future depression.

- The Adolescent Coping with Depression [CWD-A] Course. This is an evidence-based treatment intervention for actively depressed adolescents. The program also includes a separate intervention for the parents of these depressed adolescents.

- The Adolescent Coping with Stress Course [CWS] Course. This is an evidence-based group prevention intervention for youth at risk for future depression.

- A brief, individual treatment program (5 to 9 sessions) for depressed youth who also are receiving SSRI antidepressant medication is available.

# References

American Psychiatric Association (2000). *Diagnostic and Statistical Manual of Mental Disorders. Fourth Edition* (DSM-IV). Washington, DC: APA.

Castiglia, P.T. (2000). Depression in children. <u>Journal of Pediatric Health Care</u>, 14(2): 73-75.

Hamrin, V. & Pachler, M.C. (2004). Depression in children and adolescents: the latest evidence-based psychopharmacological treatments. *Journal of Psychosocial Nursing*, 42(4): 10-15.

Kaye, D.L., Montgomery, M.E., & Munson, S. (2002). *Child and Adolescent Mental Health.* Philadelphia, PA: Lippincott.

Jellinek, M., Patel, B.P., & Froehle, M. (2002). *Bright Futures in Practice: Mental Health- Vol I. Practice Guide.* Arlington, VA: National Center for Education in Maternal and Child Health.

Jellinek, M., Patel, B.P, & Froehle, M. (2002). *Bright Futures in Practice: Mental Health- Vol II. Tool Kit.* Arlington, VA: National Center for Education in Maternal and Child Health.

Melnyk, B.M., Brown, H., Jones, D.C., Kreipe, R., & Novak, J. (2003). Improving the mental/psychosocial health of U.S. children and adolescents. Outcomes and implementation strategies from the national KySS summit. *Journal of Pediatric Healthcare*, 17 (6: Supplement 1), S1- S24.

Moldenhauer, Z. & Melnyk, B.M. (in press for 2006). Assessment and management of common mental health disorders in children and adolescents. In N. Ryan-Wenger (Ed), NAPNAP/AFPNP: Core Curriculum for Pediatric Nurse Practitioners. Philadelphia, PA: Elsevier

Murphy, K. (2004). Recognizing depression in children. *Nurse Practitioner*, 29(9): 18-31.

Schapiro, N.A. (2005). Bipolar disorders in children and adolescents. *Journal of Pediatric Health Care*, 19(3): 131-141.

# Section 8
## Marital Separation and Divorce
### Bernadette Melnyk and Linda Alpert-Gillis

Section 8
Marital Separation
and Divorce

# Information for Healthcare Providers about Marital Separation and Divorce

## Quick Facts

- Divorce affects more than 1 million children every year.
- It is common for inter-parental conflict to heighten in the first year after marital separation.
- There is a wide variation in how parents respond to marital separation and divorce.

Shortly after separation, some parents experience a "honeymoon" period in which they feel relieved that a stressful marriage has ended, whereas others feel anxiety, anger/guilt, depression, exhaustion, and helplessness.

These negative feelings may result in an increase in smoking and alcohol/drug usage.

- Most adults report that their low point is one year after marital separation, with full adjustment taking 2 to 3 years.
- Evidence has supported that the 2 most important factors influencing how children deal with their parents' separation and divorce is how their parents are coping with this transition as well as the quality of parenting that they continue to receive from them.
- Discipline is a major challenge after separation (i.e., parents may treat their children as vulnerable because of guilt feelings and have difficulty setting limits), especially for the parent who has not been the primary disciplinarian.
- Divorce and its related stressors place children at short- and long-term risk for psychological, emotional, academic and behavior problems.
- Approximately one third of children adjust well, one third of children have moderate adjustment difficulties, and one third have substantial adverse outcomes.
- It is important to educate parents about the common responses that children and teens have in response to marital separation and divorce as well as what they can do to help their children cope with this transition.

# Typical Responses to Marital Separation

## Young Children

- Regression
- Irritability and restlessness
- Temper tantrums
- Sleeping difficulties
- Separation problems
- Anger
- Increased whining and crying
- Sadness
- Guilt
- Fear of abandonment
- Excessive clinging
- Withdrawal

## School-Aged Children

- Sadness
- Depression
- Longing for parent's return
- Withdrawal
- Denial
- Somatic complaints
- Parentification
- Deterioration in school performance
- Low self-esteem
- Anger
- Preoccupation with parent's
- departure from home
- Decrease in peer relations
- Shame
- Loyalty conflicts
- Reunification fantasies
- Behavioral problems

## Adolescents

- Anger
- Blaming one parent
- Attempts to gain control
- Denial
- Somatic complaints
- Low self-esteem
- Sadness
- Depression
- Loyalty conflicts
- Acting out or immature behaviors
  Parentification
- Increase in sexual activity
  and drug and alcohol usage
- Withdrawal

# Critical History-Taking Questions When a Divorce or Separation has Occurred

- Have there been any changes in your family since your last visit? (This is an essential question as parents may not disclose a marital transition unless directly asked.)
- What are the parents' and child's perceptions of the divorce?
- What have the parents told the child about the divorce?
- How are the parents and child coping with the divorce and what are their responses? Specifically, how have their emotions and behaviors changed?
- What is the parents' knowledge of the impact of divorce on their children and the typical responses that children have when adjusting to the transition?
- What changes have occurred in parenting practices and daily routines (e.g., employment, child care)?
- What are the family's other major life stressors (e.g., move to a new home, change in job, financial difficulties)?
- How much conflict between the parents is occurring, and is the child a witness to that conflict?
- What social supports do the parent and child have in place to assist them in coping with the separation and divorce?
- What is the level of involvement of the noncustodial parent?
- What is the parents' and child's mood state (e.g., anxiety, depression)? Specifically ask, on a scale of 0 to 10, "How stressed/anxious as well as depressed are you (your child) on a daily basis?"
- What is the parents' and child's current level of functioning (e.g., at work and at school)?
- What is worrying the parent and child most at this time?

## Early Interventions

- Emphasize to the parent that how they are coping with the divorce and their quality of parenting are the 2 major factors that will affect how their children adjust to the transition.
- Advise the parent to obtain counseling if he or she is feeling very anxious or depressed.
- Inform the parent that it is not helpful to set unrealistic expectations for themselves or their children and that the process of adjustment to this transition may take up to 2 to 3 years.
- Educate the parent about typical age-appropriate responses that children have to separation and divorce.
- Counsel parents about age-appropriate strategies to help their children cope with the transition.
- Provide parents with the handouts "A dozen ways to help your child deal with divorce" and "Coping with marital separation and divorce: a selected bibliography for children and parents," available in this guide.
- Advise parents to consistently reinforce to their child that: (a) the divorce is not the child's fault (as children often feel guilty about it); and (b) that they will not abandon him or her (children need this reinforcement).

---

- Encourage parents to help their children openly express their feelings about the divorce (younger children often express their feelings by talking about how their stuffed animal or puppet feels).
- Advise parents that talking to and about the other parent in negative ways will lower their child's self-esteem.
- Counsel parents on the negative effects of parental conflict.
- Encourage parents to spend special time with their child every day, even if only for 15 minutes, without interruptions, and to maintain routines.
- Assist the parent with discipline; encourage the importance of setting of limits and reinforcing them consistently. (Although he or she cannot control what happens at the other parent's home, the parent can implement limits at his or her own home.)
- Offer parents the COPE program (Creating Opportunities for Parent Empowerment), an evidence-based user-friendly program designed to assist parents in helping 3 to 7 year old children cope with divorce. The program can be obtained at www.COPEforHOPE.com.
- Provide local resources to help parents and children deal with the divorce (e.g., Parents without Partners).
- Inform the parents to contact you with any concerns or worries about their child.

Reprinted with permission from: Melnyk, B.M. & Alpert-Gillis, L.J. (1997). Coping with marital separation. Smoothing the transition for parents and children. *Journal of Pediatric Health Care, 11: 165-174.*

# Screening for Marital Transitions

Because of the major impact that marital transitions (i.e., separation, divorce, remarriage) have on families, it is very important to ask the following questions at each healthcare encounter.

**For Parents and Children/Teens:**

Have there been any changes in your family in the past year, such as marital separation/divorce or remarriage?

On a scale of 0 to 10, if 0 means "there is no fighting" and 10 means "there is a lot of fighting," how much arguing/fighting goes on in your home?

On a scale of 0 to 10, if 0 means you "have no stress" and 10 means you have "a lot of stress," how much stress is the divorce causing you?

On a scale of 0 to 10, if 0 means "not at all" and 10 means "a lot," how much is the divorce affecting your ability to work (for parents) or to do well in school (for children/teens)?

# A Dozen Ways to Help your Child Deal with Marital Separation/Divorce

1. Understand the impact of divorce on children.

Marital separation involves stressful and difficult transitions for children and parents. It is common for children to show some behavioral changes in response to such transitions. There are parenting strategies that can help you and your children cope effectively with your family situation.

2. Prepare your children for the changes involved in a divorce.

Give children information about family changes in a way they can understand Tell children in advance about the changes they are about to experience.

3. Accept children's feelings and encourage them in constructive ways.

Help your children learn to talk about their feelings and express feelings acceptable ways. When children can put their feelings into words, they are much less likely to act out inappropriately.

4. Reassure your children.

Make sure that your children know that you love them and that you will take care of them. Inform your children that you are divorcing the other parent, not them. Provide assurance that a parent's love for a child is a special kind that does not stop.

5. Allow your children to be children.

Avoid having your child take on too many adult responsibilities. Discussing family finances with them or telling them that they are now the "little man or woman of the house" can be a burden. Instead, encourage them to become involved in school activities, clubs, or hobbies that develop their own strength and abilities.

6. Give children permission to love both parents. Support your children's relationship with their other parent.

Children benefit from a positive relationship with both a consistent shedule of when children will be with each parent is very important. Also, not talking in a negative way about the other parent can allow your children a healthier relationship with both parents.

7. Problem solve together.

Talk with your children about how to make things better or more comfortable for them.

8. Work on your relationship with your children.

Set aside special time to spend with each child, doing things together such are reading, playing a game, or taking a walk.

9. Keep conflict away from your children.

Keep arguments with your former spouse as far away from your children as possible, especially if they involve verbal or physical aggression. Intense conflict between parents is likely to lead to adjustment problems in children. Do not use your children as messengers or as weapons to get back at your former spouse.

10. Maintain as much structure and predictability in your everyday routine as possible.

Children thrive on routine, including regular bedtimes, having meals together and consistent rules. Setting limits on children's inappropriate behavior helps children feel safe and communicate to them that you will provide order and control when they are not able to do so.

11. Listen to children's verbal and nonverbal communication.

Listen to what your children say and watch what they do. Remember that all children often state things indirectly. For, example, "I hate the woman you're dating" may mean "I am worried that you like her more than me."

12. Take care of yourself.

Reach out to resources such as trusted friends, family members, support groups, members of the clergy and mental health professionals. Research has emphasized the important link between parents' emotional and physical well-being and children's healthy development.

Reprinted with permission from: Melnyk, B.M. & Alpert-Gillis, L.J. (1997). Coping with marital separation. Smoothing the transition for parents and children. *Journal of Pediatric Health Care, 11:* 165-174.

# Internet Resources

## American Academy of Child and Adolescent Psychiatry
www.aacap.org
This Web site is an excellent source of information on the assessment and treatment of child and adolescent mental health disorders. Handouts for use with families (i.e., *Facts for Families*) are available on a multitude of problems, including divorce.

## KidsHealth
www.kidshealth.org
This is an outstanding Web site that contains health information for healthcare providers, parents, teens, and children. Many of the topics relate to emotions and behaviors (e.g., anxiety, fears, and depression) as well as family changes and are developmentally sensitive to specific age groups. Physicians and other healthcare providers review all material before it is posted on this Web site.

# References

Jellinek, M., Patel, B.P., & Froehle, M. (2002). *Bright Futures in Practice: Mental Health- Vol I. Practice Guide.* Arlington, VA: National Center for Education in Maternal and Child Health.

Jellinek, M., Patel, B.P., & Froehle, M. (2002). *Bright Futures in Practice: Mental Health- Vol II. Tool Kit.* Arlington, VA: National Center for Education in Maternal and Child Health.

Melnyk, B.M., Brown, H., Jones, D.C., Kreipe, R., & Novak, J. (2003). Improving the mental/psychosocial health of U.S. children and adolescents. Outcomes and implementation strategies from the national KySS summit. *Journal of Pediatric Healthcare*, 17 (6: Supplement 1): S1- S24.

Moldenhauer, Z. & Melnyk, B.M. (in press for 2006). Assessment and management of common mental health disorders in children and adolescents. In N. Ryan-Wenger (Ed), NAPNAP/AFPNP: Core Curriculum for Pediatric Nurse Practitioners. Philadelphia, PA: Elsevier

Teyber, E. (2001). *Helping Children Cope With Divorce.* New York, NY: Josey Bass Company.

# Information for Healthcare Providers about Maltreatment

## Quick Facts

- **Child abuse** is defined as the causation of a nonaccidental injury.
- **Child neglect** is defined as the omission of a child's basic needs. It is a significant cause of morbidity and mortality in children.
- About 3 million reports are filed each year on children suspected to have been abused or neglected. Out of these about 1 million are substantiated.
- Every day, 4 children in our country die of child maltreatment. Most victims are under 6 years of age.
- Domestic violence is significantly intertwined with child maltreatment. Millions of children witness domestic violence in their lifetime, doubling the risk of child maltreatment if the mother is being battered.
- Girls who are abused as children are far more likely to become victims of violence as adults.
- Boys abused as children are more inclined to commit acts of violence as adults.
- Child maltreatment tends to be repetitive and frequently will escalate over time. In many cases the abuser does not intend to hurt the child. Rather, abuse is the result of unrealistic caretaker expectations and poor coping mechanisms.
- Although abuse occurs in all aspects of society, multiple socioeconomic factors help identify children at greater risk.

## Child Risk Factors Include Children with the Following

- Fussy temperaments
- Chronic medical conditions/congenital anomalies
- Developmental disabilities
- Behavioral problems
- Children under 3 years old
- Children in foster care

## Parent Risk Factors

- Young parents
- Single parents
- Parents with a history of being abused
- Unwanted pregnancy
- Poverty or social stressors
- Substance abuse/mental illness/developmental delay
- Domestic violence

## Triggers of Abuse

- Excessive crying
- Acute illness
- Frequent nighttime awakenings
- Potty training problems
- Feeding issues
- Oppositional behavior

## Prevention Is Key

We are all aware that child maltreatment is extremely detrimental to children. As healthcare providers, it is important to focus on prevention and to recognize the risk factors early on for our patients. Advocating for our children and families is the key to prevention!

## Remember: All Healthcare Providers Are Mandated Reporters

You don't have to decide whether or not a child is being maltreated - that is the responsibility of Child Protective Services (CPS). You are mandated to report if you have a reasonable suspicion of abuse or neglect. There are certain physical or behavioral indicators that should raise a red flag about the possibility. The history must always be put together with the behavioral and physical indicators. Clearly, some of these indicators may be the result of other stressors in a child's life. Any one indicator is not definitive - it just raises questions. Many primary care providers are resistant to making CPS reports-they feel they "know" the family well and want to spare the "nice" family the aggravation of dealing with CPS - but please try to be objective and make referrals to CPS based on the history and indicators.

## Behavioral Indicators

- Mood swings including aggression, depression, anxiety, and oppositional behavior
- Suicidal ideation
- Alcohol or drug abuse
- School problems

- Poor social interactions/withdrawing
- Appetite/sleep changes
- Regression
- Provocative or sophisticated behavior
- Psychosomatic complaints (e.g., recurrent headaches, stomachaches)
- Runaway behavior
- Self-injurious behavior

**Physical Indicators**

- Bruising on the face, neck, wrists, ankles, back, genitals, thighs; bruises in the shape of a hand or object
- Bites that are too large to be a child's
- Lacerations in the mouth of an infant
- Burns that are patterned, immersion, cigarette shaped
- Any fracture occurring in a child aged 1 year or younger; fractures of the skull, spiral, rib, metaphyseal, spinal, hands/feet, or fractures in multiple stages of healing
- Head trauma with subdural hematomas, retinal hemorrhages
- Bruising, bleeding, abrasions, lesions, discharge, pain in the genital region
- Pregnancy or sexually transmitted infection - depending on age and situation
- Neglect issues (e.g., inappropriate clothing, poor weight gain, poor medical compliance, lack of appropriate supervision, poor hygiene)
- Any injury that does not fit the history

# DSM-IV Criteria for Child Maltreatment

This section includes categories that should be used when the focus of clinical attention is severe mistreatment of one individual by another through physical abuse, sexual abuse, or child neglect. These problems are included because they are frequently a focus of clinical attention among individuals seen by health professionals.

---

**Physical Abuse of a Child**
This category should be used when the focus of clinical attention is physical abuse of a child.

**Sexual Abuse of a Child**
This category should be used when the focus of clinical attention is sexual abuse of a child.

**Neglect of a Child**
This category should be used when the focus of clinical attention is child neglect.

---

# Screening Tools for Child Maltreatment

There are very few screening tools that have been scientifically tested to aid in the identification of child abuse. Currently, there are a number of studies that are looking at the feasibility of utilizing a tool for this purpose. However, there is insufficient evidence to justify screening tools to adequately predict child maltreatment. One of the main challenges for healthcare providers is how to add more questions in an already limited time period. Another major concern is how to adequately screen the parent for violence issues with the child in the room and how to screen the child for abuse issues with the parent in the room. The Edinburgh Postnatal Depression Scale or Beck Post-partum Depression Screening Scale (information about the PDSS is contained in the mood disorders section of this guide) are two scales that are currently being utilized in some pediatric practices. There is evidence to support that a mother who is depressed is at high risk for neglect and abuse of her child. The GAPS (Guidelines for Adolescent Preventive Services) form for adolescents (see Assessment and Screening section of this guide) briefly addresses abuse and may provide insight to the provider. Any of the tools that are currently being utilized for other mental health disorders also may be useful in identifying abuse and neglect. The following screening questions may be used during a visit to identify abuse and violence in the home.

## Questions for Parents

- Are you afraid of anyone in your home?
- Do you ever feel so frustrated that you fear you may hit or hurt your child?
- Are you feeling overwhelmed?
- Have the police come to your home?

## Questions for Children/Teens

- Are you afraid of anyone in your home?
- Whom could you tell if anyone has touched you in a way that made you feel not okay? Has this ever happened to you?
- What happens when your parents are angry with you?
- What happens when adults in your home are angry at each other?
- Have the police been to your home?

# Information for Parents on Child Maltreatment

## Important Facts

Child abuse and neglect is defined as causing nonaccidental injury or not providing a child's basic needs. About 3 million reports are filed every year on children that someone suspects may have been abused or neglected.

Every day, 4 children in our country die from child abuse. Most of the victims are under 6 years old. However, teenagers between the ages of 12 and 17, particularly girls, also have been victims of child abuse.

Child sexual abuse is any use of a child for the sexual gratification of an adult. This includes touching a child's genitals, making a child touch someone else's genitals, pornography, and exposing a person's genitals to a child.

Domestic violence is closely related to child abuse. Millions of children witness domestic violence every day. The risk of these children being abused doubles if the mother is being battered. Girls raised in violent homes are at risk for becoming victims of violence as they grow older, while boys are at risk for growing up to be aggressive and violent. Many times the abuser does not intend to hurt the child. Often, they are a loving parent or caregiver who loses control and has unrealistic expectations of the child. Child abuse and violence happens on every level of society. However, it tends to be more frequent in homes that have a lot of stressors.

It also is important to know that the majority of children who are sexually or physically abused are violated by someone they know.

## How You Can Protect Your Children and Adolescents

There are some behavioral signs in children that may indicate a child is being abused. However, some of these can be the result of other stressors in a child's life. Any one sign doesn't mean the child is being abused, but the presence of several of these signs should raise concern.

- Appetite changes
- Nightmares/change in sleeping habits
- Mood swings including aggression, depression, anxiety
- Suicidal ideation
- Provocative behavior
- Extreme fears
- Regression of behavior

- Alcohol/drug abuse
- School problems
- Frequent complaints of headaches and stomachaches

**In addition to behavior signs, here are some physical signs to alert you.**

- Frequent bruising, especially in a young infant or on the face, chest, back, or genitals
- Pain, extreme redness, discharge, or lesions in the genital region
- Injuries/fractures that are inconsistent with the description of the injury
- Poor weight gain, inappropriate clothing, no medical care for a child

**If you are concerned about any behavioral or physical signs of abuse, please call your primary care provider. They can guide you through the process of how to figure everything out.**

It is important to teach children about safety and protecting themselves as they get older. Here are some things that you and your family can do to prevent abuse:

- Adults must watch for signs of abuse as young children cannot protect themselves.
- Be alert to changes in their behavior and discuss it with them.
- Teach your children how and when to say "no." They need to know that they can say no if someone makes them uncomfortable or scared.
- Set privacy boundaries within your family.
- Teach children that special secrets about touching or physical harm are not okay.
- Teach children the correct names of body parts.
- Make sure to keep the lines of communication open. LISTEN AND TALK to your children and adolescents all the time. Make sure they know they can talk to you.
- Do not confuse children with the "stranger danger" concept. This message is not effective, as danger to children is greater from someone they know.
- Screen all caregivers carefully, such as babysitters, day care providers, and coaches.
- Teach your children and adolescents how to get out of a threatening situation. Make a family safety plan!
- Supervise Internet use -- many sexual predators use this to connect with children.
- Make arrangements ahead of time to be available for your children when they go out with friends. They need to know they can call you for a ride if they find themselves in an uncomfortable position or if they have used substances and feel unsafe to drive home.
- Always report anything suspicious.

**Be a parent that is involved in your children's lives. Take the time to listen to your children, which will help them to develop their sense of security. Communication is key. Also, find ways to help yourself if you are feeling stressed. Remember, your stress affects your children.**

*This handout may be photocopied (but not altered) and distributed to families. From Melnyk, B.M. & Moldenhauer, Z: The KySS™ Guide to Child and Adolescent Mental Health Screening, Early Intervention and Health Promotion, ©, 2006, National Association of Pediatric Nurse Practitioners and the NAPNAP Foundation, Cherry Hill, NJ.*

# Information for Adolescents on Child Maltreatment

## Important Facts

There are many different forms of child abuse and neglect. It can happen to any child, at any age, including adolescents. Here are some things that could be child abuse:

- An adult is hurting you physically, such as hitting you, especially if it is with an object.
- An adult is touching you in private places such as the breast or genitals, or having any form of sex with you.
- One of your friends tries to have sex with you after you have said "NO."
- A boyfriend/girlfriend can abuse you if he is physically or emotionally abusive to you.
- You don't have a warm place to stay.
- You don't receive medical care.
- There isn't enough food in the house.
- Your parents keep you out of school.
- Emotional abuse can happen if your caregivers are always mean to you and make you feel bad about yourself.

Teenagers are the group of people most often victimized in the United States. This is especially true for girls. Here are some things that you should be aware of:

- Teenage girls are the most frequent victims of sexual assault.
- More than 50% of all rape victims are under 18 years old.
- One in 4 college women have been raped or have experienced attempted rape.
- 93% of juvenile sexual assault victims knew their attacker.
- Four out of 10 sexual assaults are in the victim's home.
- Two out of 10 sexual assaults take place in the home of a friend.
- One out of 5 victims of sexual assault are male.

The impact of rape includes physical trauma, genital trauma, pregnancy, sexually transmitted infections, and psychological symptoms.

Many teenagers experience a lot of problems after being sexually abused or assaulted. These include:

- Substance abuse
- Depression and anxiety
- Difficulty with close relationships
- Suicide thoughts

- Violent behavior
- Nightmares and difficulty sleeping
- Frequent headaches and stomachaches

## How can you prevent this from happening to you

- Tell a trusted adult if someone is hurting you emotionally, physically or sexually at home.

- Tell a trusted adult if another person in your peer group is forcing you to have sex or hurting you physically.

- Never go out alone!  There is always safety in numbers.  Don't hitchhike!

- Make sure that an adult knows where you are going and with whom.

- Be careful of the Internet.  It is NEVER a good idea to meet a stranger with whom you have been communicating online.

- Don't go to parties or gatherings where there is no adult present.  Although it may sound fun and very grown up, there can be lots of activities going on that you aren't ready for, such as alcohol and drug use and sexual activity.

- Make arrangements with a trusted adult before you go out with friends to be able to call for a ride if you find yourself in an uncomfortable position.  This would also work if you have been using drugs or alcohol and feel unsafe to drive home.  Remember, **NEVER** get in a car with anyone who has been using drugs or drinking.

- Don't let food or beverages out of your sight!  Someone may tamper with it by adding drugs.

- Remember that if someone abuses or assaults you, **IT IS NOT YOUR FAULT!!**

# Information on Child Abuse and Neglect
# for School-Age Children

There are many different ways that a child your age may be abused.  Child abuse means that an older child, teenager, or adult is hurting you.  It may be one of your parents or someone else that you care about in your family or a family friend.

**Here are some things that could be child abuse or neglect**

- An adult/teenager is hitting you, biting you, or giving you burns.

- Someone is touching you in your private areas, such as your penis (where boys pee from), rectum (where you poop from), breasts, or urethra/vagina (where girls pee from).

- If they touch you over your clothes or under your clothes, it is not okay.

- It is not okay to touch you in any of your private places with their fingers, any parts of their body, or any kind of object.

- Someone shows you their private parts or asks you to touch them or shows you movies with people that have their clothes off.

- Your parent/guardians do not send you to school.

- There is no heat in your house.

- There is not enough food in your house.

- You do not have enough clothes to keep you warm.

- Your parents/guardians do not bring you to the doctor when you are sick or hurt.

**So what do you do if someone is hurting you or touching you in a way that doesn't seem right?**

**Turn over the page to find out!**

**Here are some things that you can do if someone is hurting you or touching you in a way that doesn't seem right**

- You can say **"NO"** very loudly when that person tries to touch you, and then tell an adult whom you trust.

- Tell someone whom you trust what is happening. Some ideas are teachers, school nurses, police, your doctor or nurse practitioner, other family members, or the other parent that isn't hurting you.

- If someone tells you to keep a secret about hurting or touching, that would be important to tell an adult whom you trust.

- Never get into anyone's car that you don't know very well. If someone tries to force you, yell very loudly and try to run away.

- If you get lost when you are out in public, go to a salesperson or checkout counter or security person and tell them you are lost - don't tell just anyone that you see.

- Never go out alone, and make sure a trusted adult knows where you are at all times.

- Learn your address and phone number.


**Remember that if someone is doing something to hurt you or
make you feel bad in any way, you need to TELL!!!**


**It is NEVER your fault.**


**Your body is your private area.
NOBODY has the right to touch it.**

# Internet Resources

## National Clearinghouse on Child Abuse and Neglect
www.nccanch.acf.hhs.gov

The <u>National Clearinghouse on Child Abuse and Neglect Information</u> is a service of the Children's Bureau, Administration for Children and Families, U.S. Department of Health and Human Services. The mission of the Clearinghouse is to connect professionals and concerned citizens to practical, timely, and essential information on programs, research, legislation, and statistics to promote the safety, permanency, and well-being of children and families. It collects, organizes, and disseminates information on all aspects of child maltreatment.

## Prevent Child Abuse America
www.preventchildabuse.org

Prevent Child Abuse America has led the way in building awareness, providing education, and inspiring hope for everyone involved in the effort to prevent the abuse and neglect of children. Working with chapters in 39 states and the District of Columbia, this organization provides leadership to promote and implement prevention efforts at both the national and local levels. The organization provides many local programs, prevention initiatives, and events to help to create awareness of this problem and communicate that prevention is possible. It comprises friends, professionals, volunteers, donors, and parents who are preventing child abuse and neglect before it ever starts.

## Rape, Abuse, & Incest National Network
www.rainn.org

The Rape, Abuse & Incest National Network (RAINN) is the nation's largest anti-sexual assault organization. RAINN operates the National Sexual Assault Hotline at 1.800.656.HOPE and carries out programs to prevent sexual assault, help victims and ensure that rapists are brought to justice.

## Shaken Baby Alliance
www.shakenbaby.com

The mission of the Shaken Baby Alliance is to provide support for families of shaken baby syndrome (SBS) victims (including adoptive and foster parents), advocate for justice for SBS victims, and increase SBS awareness.

# References

American Psychiatric Association (2000). *Diagnostic and Statistical Manual of Mental Disorders, Fourth Edition* (DSM-IV). Washington, DC: APA.

Kaye, D.L., Montgomery, M.E., & Munson, S. (2002). *Child and Adolescent Mental Health.* Philadelphia, PA: Lippincott.

Jellinek, M., Patel, B.P., & Froehle, M. (2002). *Bright Futures in Practice: Mental Health- Vol I. Practice Guide.* Arlington, VA: National Center for Education in Maternal and Child Health.

Jellinek, M., Patel, B.P., & Froehle, M. (2002). *Bright Futures in Practice: Mental Health- Vol II. Tool Kit.* Arlington, VA: National Center for Education in Maternal and Child Health.

Melnyk, B.M., Brown, H., Jones, D.C., Kreipe, R., & Novak, J. (2003). Improving the mental/psychosocial health of U.S. children and adolescents. Outcomes and implementation strategies from the national KySS summit. *Journal of Pediatric Health Care*, 17 (6 Supplement): S1- S24.

Scheid, J. (2003). Recognizing and managing long-term sequelae of childhood maltreatment. *Pediatric Annals*, 36: 391-401.

## Information for Healthcare Providers on Adolescent Sexuality

### Pubertal Development

### Girls

- More girls are showing signs of breast development at age 7, although traditional teaching has been that breast development before age 8 is premature. The debate about whether to lower the age of "normal" breast development to age 7 continues.
- The average age of menarche is 12 1/2 years.
- African American girls tend to develop 1 to 2 years earlier than white girls.

### Boys

- Testicular enlargement is usually the first sign of puberty in boys and occurs on average at age 11 1/2 years.
- Spermarche (onset of sperm emission) occurs on average at age 13.4 years.
- Black boys appear to enter puberty sooner than their white counterparts.

### Parent and Adolescent Sexual Development and Sexuality

- Sexuality is a normal part of childhood and adolescence, though it changes throughout.
- Parents often view sexuality as the big issue for adolescents, and one that is an uncomfortable issue.
- Parents can and should be the key in helping youngsters develop a healthy sense of their own sexuality.

### Quick Facts about Teen Sexual Behaviors

- Although teen pregnancy rates have been decreasing, the rates in the United States are still higher than in other developed countries. The decline in teen pregnancy has been attributed in part to lower rates of sexual activity (this explains about 25% of the decline), but mostly attributed to use of effective contraceptives (explains about 75% of the decline).
- Similarly, rates of sexually transmitted diseases (STDs) in teens are higher in the United States than in other countries.
- Each year, 4 million US teens contract a STD.

- Approximately 25% of new cases of HIV infection occur in teens younger than 20 years of age.
- American teens and young adults have a disproportionately high rate of STDs compared with other age groups.
- If sex is initiated during the early teen years, these teens are likely to have several sex partners during their teenage years and are less likely to use condoms.
- The majority of teenage girls have intercourse for 18 months before seeking contraception.
- Oral sex in teens is on the rise and there is a misperception that this is a safe form of sex.
- The suicide rate is approximately 3 times higher in gay and lesbian youth as a result of isolation, peer ridicule, abuse, assault, rejection by others, and lack of self-acceptance.
- Gay/lesbian/bisexual/transgender youth suicide account for 30% of all youth suicide.
- Primary care providers must talk to their adolescent patients about sexuality at every health maintenance visit and at other appropriate times.
- Many teens perceive that their providers are uncomfortable or lack communication skills to discuss sexuality adequately.
- In one study, fewer than half of primary care providers asked adolescents about sexual activity and even fewer asked questions about sexually transmitted infections, condom use, sexual orientation, number of partners, or sexual abuse (Killebrew & Garofalo, *Pediatric Annals*, 2002, p. 567)
- **TALKING TO TEENS ABOUT SEXUALITY DOES NOT PROMOTE SEXUAL ACTIVITY.**

## Role of Healthcare Providers

- Healthcare providers should begin discussions with children and parents about the changes of puberty before the onset, approximately age 7 for girls and 9 or 10 for boys - depending on race or family history of pubertal timing. By opening up the discussion in your office, parents will be more likely to continue the discussion with their children.

- Make sure that parents know that even though their older children and teens may seem uninterested in what they think, parents actually have more influence over their children than anyone else. Research shows that young people want to get information about sexuality from their parents and that young people whose parents speak to them about sexuality early before they become sexually active are more likely to delay sexual debut and be responsible when they become sexually active.

## What should the healthcare provider do when a problem is disclosed

The teen discloses that he/she is gay, bisexual or transgender:
- Ask whether the teen has disclosed this to his/her family. If yes, what was their reaction?
- Question carefully about depression and suicidality, as these teens are at higher risk. Refer for mental health services as needed.
- Provide anticipatory guidance around risks that homosexual youth may face and discuss concerns about disclosure with teens who have not disclosed to their families. Refer for mental health services as needed.
- Be familiar with resources in the community for teens and parents, such as Parents, Families, and Friends of Lesbians and Gays (www.pflag.org), Healthy Initiatives for Youth (www.hify.org), and The Human Rights Campaign (www.hrc.org), among others.

## What should the healthcare provider do when the teen discloses current or former sexual abuse or date rape?

- If the abuse is current, the provider must take the steps required legally for reporting abuse and the teen should be examined by someone certified as a sexual assault nurse/forensic examiner.
- If the abuse or rape was in the past, in addition to providing appropriate physical examination and testing, the provider must ascertain whether the teen has disclosed this before and whether or not he/she received counseling.
- The provider should reassure the teen that what happened was not his/her fault. This reassurance is a key step in providing care to the teen.
- Discuss the option of counseling.

## Legal Issues

- Most states entitle minors (younger than 18) to receive reproductive health care without parental consent or notification. Check the laws in your state.

## Evidence-Based Interventions

- PREVENTION is the key; Interventions must begin BEFORE sexual activity is initiated.

- ABSTINENCE AND PROTECTION SHOULD BE THE DUAL CONSISTENT MESSAGE.

- Most effective preventive interventions for teens are conducted in groups and use teen peer counselors.

- Conduct motivational interviewing/assess where teens are on the stages of change.

- Teach information/motivation/behavior-change strategies.

- There is a paucity of evidence on how effective interventions delivered in primary care are in reducing risky behaviors and STDs.

- Preventing easy access to confidential, healthcare services increases screening and treatment.

## Interventions in Primary Care Settings

- Discuss sexual health and sexual development (prior to adolescence).
- Discuss healthy behaviors.
- Facilitate communication between parents and children/teens.
- Conduct an annual Pap smear and STD testing on all sexually active teens.
- Use a developmental approach to the first pelvic exam. Remember, how the first pelvic exam is conducted will have an influence on further compliance with future pelvic exams.
- Guidelines and up-to-date specific treatments of STDs are available at www.cdc.gov.

# Screening Tools/Questions for Adolescent Sexuality

## Screening Questionnaires

Before taking a history, it is important to inform the adolescent that you will be asking personal questions and that you are asking these questions so you can provide the best possible care. It also is important to let the teen know that you ask these questions of all adolescents.

The number 1 reason that adolescents do not confide in their healthcare providers about their sexuality and sexual risk-taking behaviors is that they have not been assured about confidentiality.

Before beginning the interview, it is important to tell the teen that what he or she tells you is confidential between the two of you unless you are told that someone has hurt him or her or that he or she wants to hurt himself or herself. Under those circumstances, you need to tell the teen that if this type of information is disclosed, you will have to make a report to another professional.

It is of great importance that the discussion is open and nonjudgmental. The provider's role is to provide information on healthy behaviors, not to judge the behaviors of the teen. Teens are very sensitive and will not likely come back if they feel they are being judged.

The HEADSS assessment is a good instrument for taking a psychological history from adolescents. Refer to Section One for additional information about the HEADSS Assessment.

## Questions about sexual behaviors include:

- Have you ever been in a romantic relationship?  Tell me about the people you have dated.
- Have any of your relationships been sexual relationships? (Define oral, anal, and vaginal sex so that they are clear on what constitutes a sexual relationship.)
- Are your sexual activities enjoyable?
- What does the term "safer sex" mean to you?
- Do you use anything, or have you used anything in the past, to prevent infections or pregnancy?  Are/were you satisfied with your method?
- Do you use condoms?  Always?  Sometimes? Once in a while? Some people are attracted to guys, some to girls, and some to both.  What about you?
- Have you ever been forced to have sex?
- Have you ever been pregnant (or gotten a girl pregnant)?
- Have you ever been told that you have a sexually transmitted disease?

These questions were adapted from:  Goldenring, J.M. & Rosen, D.S. (2004).  Getting into adolescent heads: an essential update. *Contemporary Pediatrics*, 21: 64-90.

- The Guidelines for Adolescent Preventive Services (GAPS) Questionnaire also contains questions about sexuality.  These are similar to the HEADSS questions.  The GAPS Questionnaire can be completed by the teen while waiting to see the provider, which can save time in a hurried clinical setting. (The GAPS forms are contained in this guide under the Screening and Assessment Section).  A URL for the questionnaire is listed under Resources for Providers, below.

# Suggested Reading for Parents on Adolescent Sexuality

1. Gaffney, D. & Roye, C. (2003). Adolescent Sexuality. Kingston, NJ: Civic Research Institute.

2. Millstein, S.G., Petersen, A.C., & Nightingale, E.O. (1993). Promoting the Health of Adolescents: New Directions for the Twenty-first Century. New York, NY: Oxford University Press.

3. Roffman, D. (2001). Sex and Sensibility: The Thinking Parent's Guide to Talking Sense about Sex. Jackson, TN: Perseus Press.

4. Roffman, D. (2002). But How'd I Get in There in the First Place? Talking to Your Young Child about Sex. Jackson, TN: Perseus Press.

5. Schwartz, P., & Cappello, D. (2000) Ten Talks Parents Must Have with Their Children About Sex and Character. New York, NY: Hyperion.

6. Richardson, J., & Schuster, M. (2004). Everything You Never Wanted Your Kids to Know About Sex (But Were Afraid They'd Ask) The Secrets to Surviving Your Child's Sexual Development from Birth to the Teens. Pittsburgh, PA: Three Rivers Press.

# Internet Resources for Older Teens on Adolescent Sexuality

## The Family Project
www.familiesaretalking.org
The Family Project, which includes the Families Are Talking Web site and newsletter, is a project of the Sexuality Information and Education Council of the United States (SIECUS). This project began in 2000 to empower parents and caregivers to communicate with their children about sexuality-related issues, to provide tools to help families communicate about these issues, and to encourage parents, caregivers, and young people to become advocates on the local, state, and national levels for sexuality-related issues including comprehensive sexuality education programs in the schools.

## Go Ask Alice!
www.goaskalice.columbia.edu
This is a health question-and-answer Internet service produced by Alice! Columbia University's Health Education Program - a division of Health Services at Columbia.

## The Teen Health Initiative (THI)
http://www.nyclu.org/thi/frames/thi_frameset.html
The THI was created in 1997 under the auspices of the New York Civil Liberty Union's Reproductive Rights Project (RRP) to work to remove the barriers that prevent young people from accessing critical reproductive health services and information. The THI staff increases awareness of minors' rights to receive confidential reproductive and other healthcare.

# Internet Resources

### The Alan Guttmacher Institute (AGI)
www.agi-usa.org/
This institute is a nonprofit organization focused on sexual and reproductive health research, policy analysis, and public education.

### The Centers for Disease Control and Prevention (CDC)
www.cdc.gov/
The CDC provides a wealth of information, including outstanding educational handouts on STDs. It also has the current guidelines for STDs.

### Guidelines for Adolescent Preventive Services (GAPS) Implementation Materials
www.ama-assn.org/ama/pub/category/1981.html
This site contains multiple resources for how to implement the GAPS tools into clinical practice.

### The National Campaign to Prevent Teen Pregnancy
www.teenpregnancy.org/
Founded in February 1996, this is a nonprofit, nonpartisan initiative supported almost entirely by private donations. Its mission is to improve the well-being of children, youth, and families by reducing teen pregnancy.

### SIECUS-the Sexuality Information and Education Council of the United States
http://www.siecus.org/
This council has served as the national voice for sexuality education, sexual health, and sexual rights for almost 40 years.

### Talking with Kids about Tough Issues
www.talkwithkids.org
This is a national campaign by Children Now and the Kaiser Family Foundation. This Web site offers practical, concrete tips and techniques for talking easily and openly with young children ages 8 to 12 about some very tough issues, such as sex, HIV/AIDS, violence, drugs, and alcohol. Outstanding educational handouts for dissemination are available.

# References

Jellinek, M., Patel, B.P., & Froehle, M. (2002). *Bright Futures in Practice: Mental Health- Vol I. Practice Guide.* Arlington, VA: National Center for Education in Maternal and Child Health.

Jellinek, M., Patel, B.P., & Froehle, M. (2002). *Bright Futures in Practice: Mental Health- Vol II. Tool Kit.* Arlington,VA: National Center for Education in Maternal and Child Health.

McEvoy, M. & Coupey, S.M. (2002). Sexually transmitted infection. A challenge for nurses working with adolescents. *Nursing Clinics of North America*, 37: 461-474.

Melnyk, B.M., Brown, H., Jones, D.C., Kreipe, R., & Novak, J. (2003). Improving the mental/psychosocial health of U.S. children and adolescents. Outcomes and implementation strategies from the national KySS summit. *Journal of Pediatric Healthcare*, 17 (6: Supplement 1): S1- S24.

Russell, S.T. & Joyner, K. (2001). Adolescent sexual orientation and suicide risk: Evidence from a national study. *American Journal of Public Health*, 91: 1276-1281.

# Section 11

## Substance Abuse
### Carole Loveland-Cherry and Jane Tuttle

## Information for Healthcare Providers about Substance Abuse

### Quick Facts

- Approximately 52% of high school students report using alcohol in the past month, and 33% are involved in binge drinking.
- Approximately 25% of high school students report using marijuana in the preceding month, and 20% report a history of sniffing or inhaling intoxicating substances.
- More than one third of high school students report smoking cigarettes within the preceding month.
- Rates of substance use increase with age and are slightly higher for males and for white adolescents.
- Marijuana is the most commonly abused illicit substance.
- There has been an increase in "Ecstasy" and steroid use in recent years.
- Teens who experiment with drugs before age 15 years have a higher risk of developing substance abuse disorder than those who do not.
- Other mental health problems frequently coexist with substance use and abuse. Adolescents sometimes use substances in an attempt to treat mental health problems, such as anxiety disorders, depression, and ADHD.

### Differences between Use and Abuse

- Children/teens that use a substance on a few occasions are typically curious about "how it feels."
- Experimentation can be described as using a substance more than a few times; usually this occurs at parties or in response to peer pressure.
- Regular use is when a child/teen uses substances every few weeks or more and it begins to affect functioning.
- Abuse is extensive use that impacts daily functioning with negative consequences.
- Dependency is when a child's/teen's life revolves around getting and using substances (the child/teen can be psychologically or physiologically dependent).

## Common Signs of Abuse

- Changes in peer group
- Decrease in school performance
- Drop in school attendance
- Disciplinary actions at school
- Changes in sleep patterns
- Frequent respiratory and gastrointestinal complaints
- An acceleration in internalizing or externalizing behaviors, including stealing money or other valuables

## Risk Factors

- Peer group use of alcohol and other drugs
- Family conflict, substance abuse, and parenting problems
- Physical or sexual abuse
- Lack of other activities
- Poor coping skills
- Poor self-esteem
- Lack of connection to adults
- Mental health disorders

## Assessing Substance Use

As with other sensitive topics, it is important to ask direct questions in a nonjudgmental manner of both parents and children/teens.

Teens and parents should be interviewed separately.

See screening questions/tools for drug and alcohol use/abuse in this section of the KySS Guide.

Inform the teen you are interviewing that the information provided will be kept confidential unless he or she tells you that what is being done is jeopardizing his or her safety; in that case, you will need to inform another professional.

When confidentiality must be broken, the child/teen should be included as to how best to inform his or her parents.

Substances can be detected in the urine, serum, and saliva. Urine toxicology screens can detect most drugs for up to a few days; however, marijuana can be detected for up to 30 days after the last use.

Alcohol is only present in the urine for a few hours. This type of testing is typically more useful as a problem is being treated versus the initial diagnosis.

# Interventions

*Preventing* substance abuse is easier than *dealing with* substance abuse.

Brief interventions (e.g., motivational interviewing) can be successful for experimentation before regular use, abuse, or dependence occurs.

The 4 steps of motivational interviewing (Miller and Rollnick) include:

1. Express empathy
2. Develop discrepancy
3. Roll with resistance
4. Support self-efficacy

More information on motivational interviewing can be found in Section 13 of this Guide.

## Brief Intervention or Brief Talk Therapy from the National Institute on Alcohol Abuse and Alcoholism (NIAAA)

*The Five Essential Steps of Brief Intervention*

### Step I. Assessment and Direct Feedback

Ask questions regarding alcohol consumption. Example: Tell me about your drinking? What do you think about your drinking?"
Ask CRAFFT questions (see screening tools).
Assess medical, behavioral, and dependence problems.

### Step II. Negotiation and Goal Setting

You need to reduce your drinking. What do you think about cutting down to 1 drink instead of 2 on the occasions that you drink?

### Step III. Behavioral Modification Techniques

Establish a treatment contract through negotiation and goal setting: Apply behavioral modification techniques: "Here is a list of situations when students drink and sometimes lose control of their drinking. What do you think you can do when you are with a group of your friends who are drinking?"

### Step IV. Self-Help-Directed Bibliotherapy

Ask patients to review a self-help booklet and complete diary cards: "I would like you to review this booklet and bring it with you at your next visit. I'd also like you to write down how much you drink on these diary cards."

### Step V. Follow-up and Reinforcement

Set up a continuing care plan for nurse reinforcement phone calls and clinic visit.

Additional information about brief intervention in primary care settings is available at the National Institute on Alcohol Abuse and Alcoholism Web site at: http://www.niaaa.nih.gov/.

**Children/teens with substance use disorders need mental health evaluation and treatment.**

# DSM-IV Criteria for Substance Abuse

## FEATURES

The essential feature of substance abuse is a maladaptive pattern of substance use manifested by recurrent and significant adverse consequences related to the repeated use of substances.

## CRITERIA FOR SUBSTANCE USE

A. A maladaptive pattern of substance use leading to clinically significant impairment or distress, as manifested by 1 (or more) of the following, occurring within a 12-month period:

1) Recurrent substance use resulting in a failure to fulfill major role obligations at work, school, or home (e.g., repeated absences or poor work performance related to substance use; substance-related absences, suspensions, or expulsions from school; neglect of children or household)

2) Recurrent substance use in situations in which it is physically hazardous (e.g., driving an automobile or operating a machine when impaired by substance use)

3) Recurrent substance-related legal problems (e.g., arrests for substance-related disorderly conduct)

4) Continued substance abuse despite having persistent or recurrent social or interpersonal problems caused or exacerbated by the effects of the substance (e.g., arguments with spouse/family members about consequences of intoxication, physical fights)

B. The symptoms have never met the criteria for substance dependence for this class of substance

*Reprinted with permission and adapted from the Diagnostic and Statistical Manual of Mental Disorders, Fourth Edition, Text Revision, Copyright 2000. American Psychiatric Association.*

# DSM-IV Criteria for Substance Dependence

## DIAGNOSTIC FEATURES

The essential feature of substance dependence is a cluster of cognitive, behavioral, and physiological symptoms indicating that the individual continues use of the substance despite significant substance-related problems. There is a pattern of repeated self-administration that usually results in tolerance, withdrawal, and compulsive drug-taking behavior.
Criteria for Substance Dependence

A maladaptive pattern of substance use, leading to clinically significant impairment or distress, as manifested by 3 (or more) of the following, occurring at any time in the same 12-month period:

| |
|---|
| (1) Tolerance, as defined by either of the following:<br><br>   (a)  A need for markedly increased amounts of the substance to achieve intoxication or desired effect<br>   (b)  Markedly diminished effect with continued use of the same amount of the substance |
| (2) Withdrawal, as manifested by either of the following:<br><br>   (a)  the characteristic withdrawal syndrome for the substance (refer to criteria A and B of the criteria sets for withdrawal from the specific substances)<br>   (b)  the same (or a closely related) substance is taken to relieve or avoid withdrawal symptoms |
| (3) The substance is often taken in larger amounts or over a longer period than was intended |
| (4) There is a persistent desire or unsuccessful efforts to cut down or control substance use |
| (5) A great deal of time is spent in activities necessary to obtain the substance (e.g., visiting multiple doctors or driving long distances), use the substance (e.g., chain-smoking), or recover from its effects |
| (6) Important social, occupational, or recreational activities are given up or reduced because of substance use |
| (7) The substance use is continued despite knowledge of having a persistent or recurrent physical or psychological problem that is likely to have been caused or exacerbated by the substance (e.g., current cocaine use despite recognition of cocaine-induced depression, or continued drinking despite recognition that an ulcer was made worse by alcohol consumption) |

*Specify* if: **With Physiological Dependence:** evidence of tolerance or withdrawal (i.e., either Item 1 or 2 is present)
**Without Physiological Dependence:** no evidence of tolerance or withdrawal (i.e., neither Item 1 nor 2 is present)

*Reprinted with permission and adapted from the Diagnostic and Statistical Manual of Mental Disorders, Fourth Edition, Text Revision, Copyright 2000. American Psychiatric Association.*

# Screening Tools for Substance Abuse

Primary healthcare providers are in a unique position to identify the use and abuse of alcohol and illicit drugs by adolescents during routine office visits and offer appropriate treatment before serious harm results.

# CRAFFT Screening Test
## (J.R. Knight)

CRAFFT is a brief alcohol and drug screening test known best by its mnemonic, which is based on the first letter of keywords in the 6 easy-to-remember questions. The CRAFFT questions include questions related to the adolescents risk-taking behaviors related to alcohol and drug use, and their feelings related to their alcohol and drug use. The CRAFFT test is most valuable to clinicians who serve adolescent patients. It can assist clinicians in discriminating adolescent patients appropriate for brief office interventions from those who need prompt referral to substance abuse specialists.

The CRAFFT test was developed by John R. Knight, MD, Director of the Center for Adolescent Substance Abuse Research at Children's Hospital in Boston, in 2002. To request complimentary CRAFFT Cards, or to request permission to make copies of the CRAFFT test, please email: info@CRAFFT.org. The CRAFFT test is also available online for clinician use at: http://www.ceasar-boston.org/studies/crafft.html.

More detailed information regarding the characteristics and use of the CRAFFT screening tool is available in the following article published in the *Archives of Pediatric and Adolescent Medicine*, June 2002, available online: *"Validity of the CRAFFT Substance Abuse Screening Test among Adolescent Clinic Patients"*.

# The CAGE Questions for Alcohol Use
## (J.A. Ewing)

The CAGE is a very brief, relatively nonconfrontational questionnaire for detection of alcoholism, usually in the "have you ever" format, but it may be focused to delineate past or present. It is generally used for adults and adolescents (over 16 years). Some of the questions may not be appropriate for teens (e.g., the eye opener).

The CAGE consists of 4 items that can be administered by pencil and paper or computer self-administered or by interview. It takes less than 1 minute to administer and can be administered by a professional or technician. There is no training required for administration; it is easy to learn, easy to remember, and easy to replicate.

- Have you ever felt that you should **CUT DOWN** on your drinking?
- Have people **ANNOYED** you by criticizing your drinking?
- Do you ever feel bad or **GUILTY** about your drinking?
- Have you ever had a drink first thing in the morning to steady your nerves or get rid of a hangover (**EYE OPENER**)?

When interpreting the client's response to the CAGE questions, some general guidelines apply. A positive response to 1 question indicates a need to question further. A positive response to 2 or more questions is a strong indication that the individual has an alcohol dependence or abuse problem, and further evaluation and intervention are needed.

The original source reference for the CAGE is: Ewing, J.A. (1984). Detecting alcoholism. The CAGE questionnaire. *JAMA*, 252: 1905-7. Additional information about the CAGE can be found at: http://www.niaaa.nih.gov/publications/cage.htm and http://www.fpnotebook.com/PSY89.htm.

# Important Information for Parents on Substance Use Disorders in Children and Teens and How to Prevent Them

- Fifty-two percent of high school students admit to using alcohol in the past month, and 33% reported binge drinking (5 or more drinks at a time). One quarter used marijuana in the past month, and 20% said they had sniffed or inhaled intoxicating substances. More than one third of high school students reported smoking cigarettes within the past month.

- Rates of substance use increase with age and are slightly higher for males and for white adolescents.

- Other mental health problems (e.g., anxiety and depression) frequently coexist with substance use and abuse. Adolescents might use substances in an attempt to treat these and help themselves to feel better.

- Common signs of substance use include changes in peer group, decrease in school performance, changes in sleep patterns, frequent respiratory and gastrointestinal complaints, and an increase in behavior problems, including stealing money or other valuables.

- Risk factors:
    Peer group use of alcohol and other drugs
    Family conflict, substance abuse, and parenting problems
    Physical or sexual abuse
    Lack of other activities
    Poor coping skills
    Poor self-esteem

Children/teens with substance use disorders need evaluation and treatment:

*Substance abuse* is defined in the *Diagnostic and Statistical Manual of Mental Disorders, Fourth Edition*, as; "A maladaptive pattern of substance use leading to clinically significant impairment or distress, and manifested by 1 or more of the following, occurring within a 12-month period:

1) Recurrent substance use resulting in a failure to fulfill major role obligations at work, school, or home,
2) Recurrent substance use in situations in which it is physically hazardous,
3) Recurrent substance-related legal problems,
4) Continued substance abuse despite having persistent or recurrent social or interpersonal problems caused or exacerbated by the effects of the substance."

## Differences between Use and Abuse:

- Children/teens that use a substance on a few occasions are typically curious about "how it feels."
- Experimentation can be described as using a substance more than a few times; usually this occurs at parties or in response to peer pressure.
- Regular use is when a child/teen uses substances every few weeks or more and it begins to affect functioning.
- Abuse is extensive use that impacts daily functioning with negative consequences.
- Dependency is when a child's/teen's life revolves around getting and using substances (the child/teen can be psychologically or physiologically dependent).

**If you believe that your child is using or abusing alcohol or drugs, talk to his/her healthcare provider about it right away.**

## How to Help Prevent Substance Use in Your Child:

- Help your child learn to problem-solve and find resources to address their challenges.
- Define position on at-risk behaviors (e.g., zero tolerance for drug or alcohol use).
- Avoid double standards (e.g., "Do as I say, not as I do"), as modeling is a powerful learning mechanism.
- Don't make excuses for children/teens. (If they think there is a problem, there usually is.)
- Frequently communicate expectations to children regarding behaviors and school performance.
- Get to know your child's friends and the parents of their friends.
- Require at least a 48 hour advance notice for sleep over events as most drug parties fall together at the last minute.
- Be available to your child; take time to listen.

For more information, access www.family.samhsa.gov and www.moniteringthefuture.org

# Important Information for Teens about Alcohol and Other Drugs

- As you get older, you may find that more of your peers are trying alcohol and other drugs. Even though the dangers of alcohol and other drug use are well known, about half of high school students admit to using alcohol in the past month, and one third report binge drinking (more than 5 drinks in one sitting).

- More than one third of high school students reported smoking cigarettes within the past month. A smaller number of young people admit to using illegal drugs, such as marijuana ("pot," "grass") and cocaine. Today, we are seeing more problems in young people related to the use of "designer" drugs such as Ecstasy.

- Serious problems also happen when young people use substances (like airplane glue) that are meant for other uses, or if they take someone else's medication.

- Young people who use alcohol and other drugs often have other mental health problems (such as depression, anxiety, ADHD). Young people sometimes use substances to try to help them with the symptoms of the other mental health problem. This is **very** risky.

- You know that you or a friend may be having a problem if you or they start "hanging out" with peers who use alcohol or other drugs, have a drop in grades, or start getting into trouble due to drug or alcohol use (arrests, suspensions, etc). Any young person who begins to lose control over her or his drinking or drug use is headed for problems. Young people who begin to go out of their way to get and use drugs or alcohol, or continue to use even after there have been problems, has a substance abuse issue.

- Young people who are most at risk for alcohol and other drug use may also have problems with:

    Family conflict
    Physical or sexual abuse
    Lack of other activities
    Poor coping skills
    Poor self-esteem
    Depression

- Some young people are also worried about the alcohol or other drug use of a family member, possibly a parent.

## Help is Available.

If you are stressed about something or worried that you may have a problem with alcohol or drugs, talk to someone you trust (e.g., your parent, doctor or nurse practitioner, or someone at school).

Don't turn to alcohol or drugs as an answer to your problems; they will just make things worse.

The following Web sites might also be helpful: www.family.samhsa.gov and www.moniteringthefuture.org.

# No Drinking and Driving Contract

I, _____, promise to keep myself safe. If I or
                    Name

a friend uses any alcohol or drugs and we are driving a motor vehicle, I will

call _____ to pick me up and drive me home.
        Name of Parent/Legal Guardian


_____          _____
Signature of Adolescent                      Signature of Provider or
                                                      Parent/Guardian


_____
Date

# Internet Resources

## Al-Anon (which includes Alateen for younger members)
www.al-anon.alateen.org/
Al-Anon has been offering hope and help to families and friends of alcoholics for a long time. This Web site provides a variety of useful publications as well as information for providers.

## American Academy of Child and Adolescent Psychiatry
www.aacap.org
This Web site is an excellent source of information on the assessment and treatment of child and adolescent mental health disorders. Handouts for use with families (i.e., *Facts for Families*) are available on a multitude of problems, including substance abuse disorders.

## Center for Adolescent Substance Abuse Research (CeASAR)
www.ceasar-boston.org
CeASAR has a Web site that provides an overview of their Adolescent Substance Abuse Program. This program provides a science-based, family-oriented, and developmentally appropriate approach to adolescent treatment.

## Monitoring the Future
www.monitoringthefuture.org
Monitoring the Future is an ongoing study of the behaviors, attitudes, and values of American secondary school students, college students, and young adults. This Web site provides ongoing reports related to the study and updates on key findings.

## National Institute on Alcohol Abuse and Alcoholism (NIAAA)- Task Force on College Drinking, a branch of the National Institutes of Health.
www.collegedrinkingprevention.gov
In response to the increasingly complex issue of alcohol abuse among college students, the National Advisory Council on Alcohol Abuse and Alcoholism created the Task Force on College Drinking in 1998.

## National Institute for Drug Addiction
www.nida.nih.gov
NIDA is a branch of the National Institutes of Health. Excellent information for professionals, parents and youth is available at this Web site.

## Substance Abuse and Mental Health Services Administration (SAMHSA)
www.family.samhsa.gov
This Web site contains educational and fact sheets about a multitude of drugs and prevention programs. To join SAMHSA's "A Family Guide to Keeping Youth Mentally Healthy & Drug Free" list serve, send an email to: familyguide@listserve.health.org.

## White House Office of National Drug Control Policy (ONDCP)
www.whitehousedrugpolicy.gov/
Their Web site has a great deal of helpful information about drugs, including street terms and legislation.

# References

American Psychiatric Association (2000). *Diagnostic and Statistical Manual of Mental Disorders. Fourth Edition* (DSM-IV). Washington, DC: APA.

Kaye, D.L., Montgomery, M.E., & Munson, S. (2002). *Child and Adolescent Mental Health.* Philadelphia, PA: Lippincott.

Jellinek, M., Patel, B.P., & Froehle, M. (2002). *Bright Futures in Practice: Mental Health- Vol I. Practice Guide.* Arlington, VA: National Center for Education in Maternal and Child Health.

Jellinek, M., Patel, B.P., & Froehle, M. (2002). *Bright Futures in Practice: Mental Health- Vol II. Tool Kit.* Arlington, VA: National Center for Education in Maternal and Child Health.

Knight, J.R., Shrier, L.A., Bravender, T.D., Farrell, M., Vanderbilt, J., & Shaffer, H.J. (1999). A new brief screen for adolescent substance abuse. *Archives of Pediatric and Adolescent Medicine,* 153: 591-596.

Knight, J.R., Sherritt, L., Schrier, LA, Harris, SK, Chang, G. (2002). Validity of the CRAFFT substance abuse screening test among adolescent clinic patients. *Archives of Pediatric and Adolescent Medicine,* 156: 607-614.

Melnyk, B.M., Brown, H., Jones, D.C., Kreipe, R., & Novak, J. (2003). Improving the mental/psychosocial health of U.S. children and adolescents. Outcomes and implementation strategies from the national KySS summit. *Journal of Pediatric Healthcare,* 17 (6: Supplement 1): S1- S24.

Miller, W.R. & Rollnick, S. (2002). *Motivational Interviewing: Preparing People for Change. Second edition.* New York, NY: Guilford Press.

Tuttle, J., Melnyk, B, & Loveland-Cherry, C. (2002). Adolescent drug and alcohol use: strategies for assessment, intervention, and prevention. *Nursing Clinics of North America,* 37: 443-460.

# Information for Healthcare Providers about Violence

## Quick Facts

- Police arrest a child/teen for a violent crime every 5 minutes.
- Homicide is the second leading cause of death in teens.
- 15% of all spinal cord injuries are a result of intentional trauma.
- Gun violence takes a child/teen's life every 3 hours.
- Youths under 14 are committing an increasing number of serious crimes.
- Between 1988 and 1997, the number of delinquency cases involving females under age 16 years increased by 89%, while the number of cases involving females 16 years and older increased by 74%.
- The number of child delinquents entering the judicial system is increasing, and since these children tend to have longer criminal careers than juveniles who become delinquent at a later age, they constitute a disproportionate threat to public safety and property.
- Crime by girls is rising at drastic rates; murders by girls have risen 64%.

## Risk Factors for Violence

The National Center for Injury Prevention and control (NCIPC) identified several factors that place youth at risk for violence and categorized these factors into 4 clusters: individual, family, peer/school, and neighborhood. These risk factors are listed below, along with others from other organizations.

## INDIVIDUAL

- History of early aggression/antisocial behaviors
- Beliefs supportive of violence
- Poor cognitive development
- Social cognitive deficits
- ADHD
- Bipolar disorder
- Lead exposure

- Age of first contact with police
- Out of home placement
- Child in need of supervision status
- Temperament misfit (with parents)
- Brain injury

## FAMILY

- Poor monitoring or supervision of children
- Child abuse
- Family violence/partner abuse
- Divorce
- Parental psychopathology
- Familial antisocial behavior
- Teen parenthood
- Parental drug/alcohol abuse
- Poor emotional attachment to parents or caregivers
- Large family size
- Developmental disability of any family member

## PEER/SCHOOL

- Associating with peers engaged in this risk or problem behavior
- Low commitment to school
- Academic failure
- Peer rejection
- Failure to bond to school
- Victim of bullying

## NEIGHBORHOOD

- Poverty and diminished economic opportunity
- High levels of transience and family disruption
- Exposure to violence
- Concentration of delinquent peer groups
- Access to weapons

### Assess for Violence Warning Signs

Recognizing the following warning signs betters the chance of detecting the potential for violence in children as young as toddlers. For some children, combinations of behaviors and events may lead to violence.

- Fire setting
- Animal cruelty
- Excessive tantrums

- Gradual withdrawal from social contacts, and eventually complete withdrawal
- Expresses feelings of isolation and being alone
- Expresses feelings of being rejected
- Irrational beliefs and ideas
- Fascination with weaponry or explosives
- Unreciprocated romantic obsession
- Drastic change in belief system
- Family or fellow students feel fear because of your child
- Violence toward inanimate objects
- Sabotages projects or equipment
- History of being a victim of violence, including physical and sexual abuse, at home, in school, or in the community
- Low interest in school
- Expresses violence in drawings or writings; listens to music with violent themes
- When doing school projects, displays "dark side" that shows anger or frustration
- Demonstrates patterns of impulsive and chronic hitting, intimidating and other bullying behaviors
- History of being bullied
- History of disciplinary problems
- Past history of violent or overt behavior, including fire setting, vandalism, lying and cheating
- Intolerance to differences when doing school projects; prejudicial attitudes toward others based on race, ethnicity, religion, language, gender, sexual orientation, ability, or physical appearance
- Inappropriate access to firearms
- Brings weapon to school
- Increased risk-taking behaviors

## Warning Signs of Imminent Violence

These signs indicate that a child is dangerously close to behaving violently and require immediate action. The safest action would be to contact police immediately.

- Serious physical fighting with peers or a family member
- Severe property destruction
- Severe rage for apparently minor reason
- Possession or use of firearms or other weapons
- Detailed plan to commit a violent act

Two of the warning signs, **fire setting and animal cruelty**, consistently correlate with violence toward humans. In a horrifying and recent example, Kip Kinkel, the 15-year-old from Springfield, Oregon, who was accused of killing his parents and two fellow students, bragged about stuffing firecrackers into cats' mouths.

Watch for a drastic change in a child's belief system, irrational beliefs, feelings of isolation or rejection, unreciprocated romantic obsession, fire setting, vandalism, a fascination with weaponry or explosives and intolerance to differences or prejudicial attitudes.

Potentially violent children may also gradually withdraw from social contacts. Other signs include: family or peers feeling fear because of the child, violence toward inanimate objects, sabotaging of projects or equipment, violence in drawings or writings, and an obsession with music with violent themes.

**Children with conduct disorder (CD):**

- Seem to be unable to correctly "read" other people.
- Instead, they misunderstand others' intentions, usually believing that others are threatening them or putting them down.
- Tend to react to these presumed threats or put-downs with aggression, with little show of feeling or remorse.
- Do not tolerate frustration well.
- Tend to behave recklessly with no regard for normal safety issues (including safe sex).
- Frequently threaten suicide - threats that should be taken seriously.

Males with CD tend to fight, steal, and participate in acts of vandalism, such as fire setting.

Females with CD lie and run away and become involved in severe sexual acting-out behavior, including prostitution.

Both males and females with CD are at very high risk of substance abuse and have severe difficulties getting along in school.

# DSM-IV Criteria for Conduct Disorder

## DIAGNOSTIC FEATURES

The essential feature of conduct disorder is a repetitive and persistent pattern of behavior in which the basic rights of others or major age-appropriate societal norms or rules are violated. It is diagnosed when a child seriously misbehaves by exhibiting aggressive or nonaggressive behaviors against people, animals or property that may be characterized as belligerent, destructive, threatening, physically cruel, deceitful, disobedient, or dishonest. This may include stealing, intentional injury, and forced sexual activity.

A. A repetitive and persistent pattern of behavior in which the basic rights of others or major age-appropriate societal norms or rules are violated, as manifested by the presence of 3 (or more) of the following criteria in the past 12 months, with at least 1 criterion present in the past 6 months:

### Aggression toward People and Animals:

(1)  Often bullies, threatens, or intimidates others

(2)  Often initiates physical fights

(3)  Has used a weapon that can cause serious physical harm to others (e.g., a bat, brick, broken bottle, knife, gun)

(4)  Has been physically cruel to people

(5)  Has been physically cruel to animals

(6)  Has stolen while confronting a victim (e.g., mugging, purse snatching, extortion, armed robbery)

(7)  Has forced someone into sexual activity

### Destruction of Property

(8)  Has deliberately engaged in fire setting with the intention of causing serious damage

(9)  Has deliberately destroyed others' property (other than by fire setting)

### Deceitfulness or Theft

(10) Has broken into someone else's house, building, or car

(11) Often lies to obtain goods or favors or to avoid obligations (i.e., "cons" others)

(12) Has stolen items of nontrivial value without confronting a victim (e.g., shoplifting, but without breaking and entering; forgery)

| Serious Violations of Rules |
| --- |
| (13) Often stays out at night despite parental prohibitions, beginning before age 13 years |
| (14) Has run away from home overnight at least twice while living in parental or parental surrogate home (or once without returning for a lengthy period) |
| (15) Is often truant from school, beginning before age 13 years |

| |
| --- |
| B. The disturbance in behavior causes clinically significant impairment in social, academic, or occupational functioning. |

| |
| --- |
| C. If the individual is age 18 years or older, criteria are not met for antisocial personality disorder. |

| |
| --- |
| *Specify* type based on age at onset: |
| **Childhood-Onset Type:** onset of at least 1 criterion characteristic of conduct disorder prior to age 10 years |
| **Adolescent-Onset Type:** absence of any criteria characteristic of conduct disorder prior to age 10 years |
| **Unspecified Onset Type:** age at onset is not known. |
| *Specify* severity: |
| **Mild:** few if any conduct problems in excess of those required to make the diagnosis and conduct problems cause only minor harm to others |
| **Moderate:** number of conduct problems and effect on others intermediate between "mild" and "severe" |
| **Severe:** many conduct problems in excess of those required to make the diagnosis, or conduct problems cause considerable harm to others |

# DSM-IV Criteria for Oppositional Defiant Disorder

## Diagnostic Criteria for Oppositional Defiant Disorder

A. A pattern of negativistic, hostile, and defiant behavior lasting at least 6 months, during which 4 (or more) of the following are present:

    (1) Often loses temper

    (2) Often argues with adults

    (3) Often actively defies or refuses to comply with adults' requests or rules

    (4) Often deliberately annoys people

    (5) Often blames others for his or her mistakes or misbehavior

    (6) Is often touchy or easily annoyed by others

    (7) Is often angry and resentful

    (8) Is often spiteful or vindictive

*Note:* Consider a criterion met only if the behavior occurs more frequently than is typically observed in individuals of comparable age and developmental level.

B. The disturbance in behavior causes clinically significant impairment in social, academic, or occupational functioning.

C. The behaviors do not occur exclusively during the course of a psychotic or mood disorder.

D. Criteria are not met for conduct disorder, and, if the individual is age 18 years or older, criteria are not met for antisocial personality disorder.

# Information for Healthcare Providers on Bullying and Gangs

- About 60% of bullies end up in the criminal justice system before they reach the age of 30, and victims have been known to retaliate in a fierce manner - most of the school shooters were bullied.

- Bullies may develop conduct disorders and delinquent behaviors during their teen years, as well as serious antisocial and criminal behavior in adulthood.

- Some bullies behave in an active, outgoing, aggressive manner, using brute force or open harassment. They reject rules and rebel to feel superior and secure.

- Others behave in a more reserved manner, not wanting to be recognized as tormentors. They control with soft-talk, saying the "right thing at the right time," and by lying, and they draw their sense of power carefully through cunning, manipulation, and deception.

- The two types may seem different, but they have the same underlying characteristics -- interest in their own pleasure, desire for power over others, willingness to manipulate others to get what they want, and the inability to see things from another's perspective.

- Bullies appear to derive gratification from inflicting injury and suffering on others. They have little to no empathy, and often defend their actions by saying that their victims provoked them. Regardless of their intelligence level, bullies usually do poorly in school and don't have good connections to their teachers. They have a hard time solving problems without violence.

- Bullies seem to have little anxiety and strong self-esteem. Contrary to popular belief, there is little evidence to support the idea that bullies victimize because they feel bad about themselves. Instead, they demonstrate inflated self-images with a need to dominate.

## Identifying Bullies

- It is more difficult to detect bullies than victims since bullies are adept at hiding their mistreatment of others and because they believe that the victims deserved what they got. Parents may have no idea that their child is bullying until a teacher or another parent confronts them about it. Bullies may act cocky, arrogant and self-assured, and they may have difficulty accepting authority. When asked about bullying, they are apt to be condescending about responding to questions.

- Garrity and Baris recommend that providers ask all children, "What do you do when others pick on you?" Bullies do not admit to even occasional confrontation with other children. Since most lack empathy, they also tend to appear pleased or amused when providers ask them how they feel about other children getting hurt.

Source: Garrity, C.B. and Baris, M.A. (1994). Caught in the Middle: Protecting the Children of High-Conflict Divorce. Jossey-Bass, Inc. Publishers, San Francisco, CA.

# Interventions

- Professionals must confront bullies and their parents about the bullying behaviors. This undertaking may be difficult as both parent and child may be reluctant to admit to bullying. Professionals should avoid arguments and advise parents that this behavior will have negative consequences on their child's future.

- Like victims, bullies benefit from learning appropriate social skills. Thus, they, also should be encouraged to participate in small group activities, preferably with older children, so that they can engage in cooperative tasks. Adult supervision is warranted during these group activities, and bullies should be reinforced each time they engage in pro-social or caring behaviors. The latter enables them to learn more positive ways to gain attention and affection.

- Professionals can work with the parents to help them learn ways to demonstrate caring and affection toward their children, as well as ways to develop more consistent and appropriate disciplinary measures. Parents should be encouraged to become more involved with community activities and other parents. If the child demonstrates significant bullying behavior or signs of a conduct disorder, referral to a mental health professional is appropriate.

## Gangs

- When teens become involved in gangs, they have higher incidences of violent and delinquent behaviors than when they are not active in a gang. Gang violence is intense, often resulting in injury and death.

- Gang problems have escalated since the 1960s, with most gangs being composed of males with similar ethnic and racial backgrounds. Ethnic conflict is associated with the emergence of gangs in certain communities, but most gang conflict occurs between gangs of the same ethnicity.

- Gang violence is no longer just an inner-city problem. Every day, more and more teens turn toward gangs to seek a "family." Many others are intimidated into joining gangs to avoid continued harassment, and still others join to get protection from other gangs. Gang members are getting more multiethnic, more youthful - children join gangs as young as 14, and sometimes even younger, and are more likely to have female members.

- Gangs tend to have a leader or group of leaders who give orders and enjoy the fruits of the gang's labors. Gang bangers (gang members) wear their "colors," certain types of clothing, tattoos, brands, or likewise imprint their gang's name, logo, or other identifying marks on their bodies. Many gangs adopt specific hairdos and communicate through hand signals and graffiti. Organized graffiti is one of the first ways to know that a gang is taking hold in your community. Experts use graffiti to track gang growth, affiliation, and membership information.

# The "Three R's" Have a Whole New Meaning in Gang Mentality

- **REPUTATION/REP** is a critical concern to gang bangers. The rep extends to each individual and the gang as a whole. Gang bangers gain status by having the most "juice" (power), based largely on one's rep. The manner in which one gains juice is important, so many members embellish their past gang activities to impress the listener, freely admitting to crimes. To even so much as gain membership, a person must be "jumped in" by being "beaten down" until the leader calls for it to end. Afterwards, they all hug each other to further the "G thing," an action that bonds members together. Young members frequently talk of this fellowship as the reason they joined the gang.

- **RESPECT** is something that they carry to the extreme, for each member, the gang, their territory, and various other things, real or perceived. Some gangs require that members always show disrespect ("dis") for rival gangs through hand signals, graffiti, or a simple "mad dog" or stare down. If a member fails to dis a rival, causing a violation to her fellow posse (gang members), she will be "beaten down" by her own gang as punishment.

- **REVENGE/RETALIATION** shows that no challenge goes unanswered in gang culture. Many drive-by shootings follow an event perceived as a dis. Typically a confrontation takes place between a gang set and a single rival gang banger. The gang banger leaves, only to return with his "home boys" to complete the confrontation and keep his rep intact.

## Warning Signs of Gang Involvement (many of these can signal other problems as well, such as drug abuse)

- Admits to being in gang
- Obsesses with one particular color or logo
- Wears excessive distinct jewelry; wears it on one side of the body
- Obsesses with "gangsta" music
- Withdraws from family
- Associates with undesirables
- Develops a strong desire for privacy
- Uses hand signals at home
- Has physical signs of being beaten and lies about events surrounding the injuries
- Wears peculiar drawings or language on books or hands
- Has unexplained cash or goods
- Uses drugs and alcohol

## Healthcare Needs of Juvenile Offenders

- Juvenile offenders have the same health maintenance needs of their non-offender peers. In addition, these children need substantial psychosocial interventions for themselves and families.

- Many of these children have conditions that may have resulted from parental neglect, mental health disorders, or physical, drug or sexual abuse; others suffer from the consequences of early sexual activity, violence, weapon use, and gang involvement. Detained youths have higher rates of depression and suicide than the general population.

- Delinquent youths are also often disenfranchised from traditional healthcare services in the community. Thus, special attention should be focused: immunization status, dental care, developmental and psychosocial issues, and establishing a plan of continued healthcare.

- All children should be evaluated for emergent, acute, and chronic conditions. Detained juvenile offenders should receive a health screening upon arrival or within 24 hours to rule out emergent needs, contagious conditions, and the need to continue current medications.

- A complete assessment and health maintenance examination with necessary interventions should be performed within 3 to 7 days. Since early sexual activity, sexual abuse, and sexual offending are all associated with delinquency; STD screening should be performed when appropriate. Young post-pubertal females should also be screened for the possibility of pregnancy.

- Juvenile offenders should receive mental healthcare in a timely manner to meet their acute and chronic emotional conditions. All children should be assessed for suicidal ideation, and precautions must be implemented for those children at risk. Psychological counseling, drug cessation programs, anger management programs and parenting classes should be available, as should appropriate education. Some children may require psychotropic medication, and provisions need to be made to provide ongoing evaluation, as standing orders for their administration may be considered inappropriate

- Detention can present a unique opportunity to address the basic health needs of these children and provide health education. However, factors can impede this process. The provision of healthcare in these facilities is multifaceted, with the potential for conflict of interest regarding custody versus care issues. Juveniles who are released and those who are not detained, easily fall through the cracks with their healthcare neglected.

## Assessing Known Juvenile Offenders

- Perform a comprehensive exam that includes a complete history and physical, with a neuropsychiatric assessment, to monitor for the possibilities of underlying neurological and psychiatric disorders, including cranial lesions, ADHD, bipolar disorder, and substance abuse.

- Laboratory evaluation should rule out lead poisoning and hyperthyroidism, which may manifest in behavioral problems. Since many of these children come from violent families, each should be carefully evaluated for signs of abuse with radiographic studies for suspicious injuries and trauma and laboratory studies to rule out STDs when sexual abuse is suspected. Toxicology studies may be warranted to assess for substance abuse.

*Adapted from the American Academy of Pediatrics Committee on Adolescence, 2001; Society for Adolescent Medicine Ad Hoc Committee Juvenile Justice Special Interest Group, 2000.*

# Teach Parents How to Raise Nonviolent Children

## Explain the Difference between Normal and Abnormal

All children behave in a negative manner at some time or another, and parents need to be able to differentiate behaviors that are appropriate for a child's age (imaginary warfare during the school-age years) from those that are not (biting after age 2). Although it is not unusual for children to exhibit some aggressive behaviors, it is socially unacceptable. Children still need limits, and parents, with your guidance, can teach and instill them.

## Encourage Parents to Provide Plenty of Love and Attention

Lack of attention causes increased aggression and reduces the ability to respond to or give affection, placing children at risk for becoming hostile, difficult, and hard to manage. Children need attention, and they manage to get it, even if it means being disruptive or obnoxious. When children feel rejected or unappreciated, they typically resort to misbehavior, which unfortunately leads to further inattention and even rejection.

You can help busy parents with time management and prioritizing skills, and encourage parents to carry out family meetings, get-togethers, and family meal times. You can also reinforce the need for parents to openly demonstrate their love and affection by telling their children they love them, hugging their children, and providing a safe, secure and nurturing home.

## Foster Positive Self-Esteem

Children with positive self-esteem typically have an easier time handling conflicts and resisting negative pressures. By contrast, children with low self-esteem feel overwhelmed by life and put themselves down or lose their temper, pick fights, blame others, constantly find fault, and take pleasure in other people's troubles.

Encourage parents to accept and praise their children for who they are, not what they do. Parents should avoid criticism, shame and comparisons, and acknowledge a child's right to have his own feelings, friends, opinions and activities. Parents should also participate in their children's lives and encourage them, without pressuring them into constructive activities before they are ready. Most importantly, parents must model their own healthy self-esteem. If parents are overly critical, pessimistic, or unrealistic about their abilities and limitations, their children will imitate them and do likewise.

## Encourage Parents to Talk *With* Their Children, Not *at* Them

Families with poor communication skills are at higher risk for raising violent children. Support and promote active listening, honesty, and reliability. Teach basic communication skills, such as talking at the child's eye level, as well as age-specific techniques and the importance of touch, a powerful communication tool.

## Enforce the Importance of Parental Supervision

A critical factor in teen violence is lack of parental supervision, particularly lack of knowledge of children's whereabouts; activities, and friends. Children with minimal parental monitoring have higher levels of problem behaviors than children with proper monitoring. Parents need to know where their children are, what they are doing, and whom they are with. They should avoid leaving young children home alone and encourage older children to participate in adult-supervised after-school activities or community programs.

## Aid Parents in Setting Limits

Children misbehave to get attention, assert power, be defiant, or act out frustrations, anger, depression or pain. They misbehave when rules are not clear or consistently applied. Therefore, parents need to set limits through effective discipline. Effective discipline takes place all the time, not just when children are naughty. It is an entire system of attitudes, instructions, models, rewards, and consequences designed to help children learn how to control their behavior. Discipline is not the same as punishment. Discourage corporal punishment, since research shows that it is demeaning, potentially harmful, and ineffective as a disciplinary measure. Teach parents how to use effective measures such as timeouts and consequences, and emphasize that parents can say "no" whenever necessary.

## Teach Responsibility

In 1970, a White House conference on youth voiced the need for children to be involved in genuine responsibilities at home and in school so they can learn to deal constructively with personal and social problems. When children have a number of responsibilities, they learn how to establish priorities and organize their time. Encourage parents to have their children participate in household chores and community service, instruct them to teach their children the difference between right and wrong, and demonstrate that behaviors, both good and bad, have consequences.

## Assist Parents in Teaching Problem-Solving and Decision-Making Skills

Children encounter problems on a regular basis, and, like decisions, some are simple and others are complex. Their approach to the problem will be based on the nature of the problem (simple vs. complex), their experience with problem solving, their mental ability, and the alternative or option chosen to solve the problem. Without effective problem management techniques, some children may withdraw and others may become aggressive. Encourage parents to foster young children's problem-solving abilities through fantasy play and older children's abilities by incorporating age-appropriate decisions (problems), such as planning what to wear for the week.

## Help Parents Help Their Children Minimize and Manage Stress

Stress overload can cause children to be withdrawn, depressed, and suicidal. It can also make them irritable, disobedient, and uncooperative. Parents need to first realize that today's children are considerably stressed due to world events and the stressors of everyday living and development. Assist parents in recognizing their child's stressors, creating ways to minimize those stressors, and utilizing stress management skills, such as hobbies, humor, relaxation techniques, and pet therapy. Encourage parents to foster healthy nutrition, exercise, and rest, since these serve as the foundation of stress management.

## Foster Anger and Conflict Management

Children with self-control and conflict management skills are respected by others and become role models, whereas children who lack self-control and appropriate conflict management skills resort to violence as an easy way to win disagreements. Children should learn to recognize their own angry feelings, express anger nonviolently, communicate anger in a positive way, calm themselves, problem-solve, remove themselves from angry situations, and avoid becoming a victim of someone else's anger. Since conflict is inevitable, children need to develop conflict resolution skills. Conflict resolution involves negotiation, mediation, or consensual decision-making. When conflicts are resolved constructively, both sides win.

## Teach Tolerance

People of color comprise about one third of all US citizens. Despite efforts and evolution, prejudice, discrimination, and hatred continue and can lead to violence. Hate crimes are acts of violence committed against people because of their ethnicity, religion, or sexual orientation. Parents can battle these crimes by fostering an understanding, tolerance, and appreciation of the differences among people.

## Enforce Family Values

Values influence behavior, both consciously and unconsciously. If children lack moral integrity, they show little regard for the rights and property of others, and they are unable to judge behavior as right or wrong. Values are learned, and if they are not taught at home, values will be absorbed elsewhere, even those that are undesirable. Children need to see and hear family values regularly, and to encourage nonviolence, the values should include: honesty and trustworthiness; loyalty; responsibility; self-discipline; independence; generosity; selflessness; empathy; compassion; tolerance; genteelness; a concern for justice; respect for self and others; courtesy; mercy; and the courage of one's convictions.

## Minimize the Effects of Peer Pressure

Peer pressure can lead to violence when children associate with peers who engage in high-risk or problem behavior. This is especially true for teenagers, who feel the need to conform to the norms of the group, and children with low self-esteem, who are the most vulnerable to negative peer pressure.

Parents can start by knowing their children's friends and their friends' parents. Knowing each other's values and rules can often stop problems before they begin. Parents can also acknowledge that a child's desire to be part of a group does not obligate them to give in to his or her every desire. But they should choose battles wisely by compromising on the minor issues, such as hairstyles and pierced ears, and by holding firm on the major issues, such as shoplifting, alcohol or drug use.

## Instruct Parents to Monitor Their Children's Media Usage

The American Academy of Pediatrics recently released a statement linking violent TV, movie, and video game images with an increase in violent behavior in children. Media violence can promote aggressive and antisocial behavior, desensitize viewers to future violence, and increase viewers' perceptions that they live in a dangerous world.

Encourage parents to minimize their children's exposure to violent media (particularly video games where the game-player is the "killer"); utilize media ratings guidelines; actively supervise their children's media usage; remove televisions and computers from children's bedrooms; set limits; and promote alternate activities, especially reading. Parents can also utilize parental controls measures, such as V-Chip technology for televisions and filtering software for computers, to block children's access to undesirable programming. However, since children tend to be more computer literate then their parents, they can usually override most control measures. Nothing works better than parental supervision.

## Help Parents Keep Their Children Away From Drugs

Teens under the influence of drugs, especially alcohol, are more likely to commit acts of violence than teens who do not use drugs. Parents need to be aware of the types of drugs available, including inhalants and club drugs, and need to realize that no one is immune to drug and alcohol problems. To prevent children from abusing alcohol and drugs, parents should start talking to their children about drugs at an early age and continue open communication throughout their development. Encourage parents to set an example and to set standards and limits on the use of alcohol and drugs in their households.

## Keep Children Away From Guns

Eighty-two percent of all homicides by 15- to 19-year-olds are committed with firearms. Since gun-play references are abundant in the media and children are exposed to guns in store windows and at home or in the homes of friends, it is impossible to completely gun-proof a child. Therefore, you must assess every child's accessibility to guns. Teach parents to instruct their children about what to do if they encounter a gun and encourage safety courses for children who utilize guns for sport.

## Empower Parents to be Responsible Role Models

Children learn best by what they see, not what they hear, and parents serve as their most important role models. Therefore, you must convince parents to act responsibly by demonstrating healthy self-esteem, being tolerant, and by managing problems in a nonviolent manner.

## Urge Parents to Get Involved

Parents should get involved in their child's school, the school's violence prevention program, and community activities. They can also support social and legislative changes that minimize youth violence. Involved parents send a strong, positive message to their children, demonstrating their commitment to education and decreasing the possibility that their children will engage in risk-taking behaviors.

## Decrease Bullying Behaviors

Bullies can grow up to be criminals, while victims can become violent themselves, as evidenced in several recent school shootings. Bullying is a nationwide problem, and school size, racial composition, and setting do not seem to be factors in predicting its occurrence. Thus, you should evaluate all children for bullying, whether bully or victim, as part of routine yearly assessment and when the presenting complaint (school phobia, somatic complaints) warrants this evaluation. Empower parents to help victims stand up to bullying and report the problem to the proper authorities, and assist parents of bullies in receiving proper counseling for their children.

## Teach Parents about the Warning Signs of Violence

Parents need to be aware of the warning signs of violence. Teach parents about both warning signs and signs of imminent violence, preferably with an accompanying handout, so that they can recognize potential problems in their children and children who influence them.

## Enable Parents to Get Help When Needed

Counseling is warranted once children deviate from the expected norm and engage in problematic behavior. Healthcare providers can first assist parents in recognizing that a problem exists, and then assist them in finding an appropriate therapist. As primary care providers, healthcare providers continue to support families during the counseling process and act as their liaison to the counselor and the school.

*From: Muscari, M. (2002). Not My Kid: 21 Steps to Raising a Nonviolent Child. Scranton, PA: University of Scranton Press. www.scrantonpress.com.*

# Screening for Violence

Providers should screen all children for violent and other antisocial behavior during wellness visits and during episodic visits where manifestations suggest the possibility of these behaviors. Questions regarding vandalism, habitual stealing, fighting, and animal cruelty can be integrated, along with questions regarding inappropriate sexual behavior, into the psychosocial history.

**Key Screening Questions**

**Questions for Parents:**

What discipline methods do you use for your child?
Do you have guns in the home?
Have there been stressful events your family is dealing with recently?

**Questions for Children and Youth:**

What do you do when you get angry?
Has anyone done anything to you that you didn't want them to do or that you didn't like?
Do you feel safe (at home, at school, in your community)?
How have the events of the world affected your family?

**Available Questionnaires for Violence:**

**GAPS (parent and teen forms)** (both forms are in this Guide)

The **Pediatric Symptom Checklist**, contained in this Guide, can identify a child at potential risk for violence or conduct/oppositional defiant problems.

# Information for Parents on How to Raise a Nonviolent Child

- ## Know the Difference Between Normal and Abnormal Behaviors & Emotions

All children behave in a negative manner at some time or another, and parents need to be able to tell the difference between behaviors that are appropriate for a child's age (imaginary warfare during the school-age years) from those that are not (biting after age 2). Although it is not unusual for children to show some aggressive behaviors, it is socially unacceptable. If your child shows these types of behaviors, it is important to set limits on them.

- ## Provide Your Child with Plenty of Love and Attention

Lack of attention causes increased aggression in children and places children at risk for becoming hostile, difficult, and hard to manage. Children need attention, even if only 15 to 20 minutes of special time with you every day. Tell your children you love them often, and provide them with a safe and secure home.

- ## Foster Positive Self-Esteem

Children with positive self-esteem typically have an easier time handling conflicts and resisting negative pressures. Praise your children often. Catch your children being good.

- ## Talk *With* Your Child, Not *at* Him or Her

Families with poor communication skills are at higher risk for raising violent children. Teach your children good, basic communication skills.

- ## Supervise your Child Closely

A critical factor in teen violence is lack of parental supervision, especially not knowing the whereabouts of children. Children with minimal parental monitoring have higher levels of problem behaviors than children with proper monitoring. Always know where your child is, with whom, and what they are doing.

- ## Set Limits with your Child

Children misbehave to get attention, assert power, or act out their frustration, anger, depression or pain. They misbehave when rules are not clear or consistent. Therefore, parents need to set limits and make sure that their children understand them. Discipline is not the same as punishment; it is teaching children what behaviors are acceptable and not acceptable. Time out as a method of discipline works well for younger children. Appropriate consequences for negative behaviors in older children and teens might include not allowing them to watch TV, play computer games, or spend time with a friend. Be consistent in setting limits with your child.

- **Teach Responsibility**

When children have a number of responsibilities, they learn how to establish priorities and organize their time. Have your child help with household chores and do some community service activities.

- **Teaching Your Child How to Problem-Solve and Make Decisions**

Encourage your child to problem-solve through play if he or she is younger. Older children should be encouraged to make age-appropriate decisions, , such as planning what to wear for the week.

- **Help Your Child to Decrease Stress**

Stress overload can cause children to be anxious, withdrawn or depressed.
Help your child to recognize signs of stress and develop ways to deal with stress (e.g., hobbies, humor, relaxation techniques, and pet therapy). Exercise also is a wonderful outlet for stress in children. Remember, your level of stress affects your child.

- **Help Your Child to Deal with their Anger in Positive Ways**

Teach your child how to recognize their own angry feelings, express anger
in positive ways, and learn positive ways for dealing with their anger (e.g., counting to 10; blowing the anger away, writing in a journal, exercising)

- **Teach Tolerance**

Help your child to understand and appreciate differences among people.

- **Enforce Family Values**

Share your values with your child regularly (e.g., honesty, compassion, self-discipline).

- **Minimize the Effects of Peer Pressure**

Know your child's friends and tell your child that being part of a group does not require them to give in to their every desire. Choose battles wisely by compromising on minor issues, such as hairstyles and pierced ears, and by holding firm on the major issues, such as shoplifting, alcohol or drug use.

- **Monitor What Your Child Watches and the Games He/She Plays**

Do not allow your children to watch violent shows or play violent video games. Studies have shown that watching violence can lead to an increase in violent behavior.

- **Keep Your Child Away from Alcohol and Drugs**

Teens under the influence of drugs, especially alcohol, are more likely to commit acts of violence than teens who do not use drugs. Start talking to your child about alcohol and drugs at an early age. Set a zero tolerance for their use.

- **Keep Guns Away from Your Child**

Do not keep guns in your home. If guns are in the home, they must be kept locked away in safe storage. Teach your child what to do if they come across a gun.

- **Be a Responsible Role Model for Your Child**

Children learn best by what they see, not what they hear, and parents serve as their most important role models. Therefore, it is important for you to show your child a healthy self-esteem and healthy ways to handle life's challenges.

- **Get Involved in Your Child's School and Activities**

Involved parents send a strong, positive message to their children, and decrease the change that their children will engage in risk-taking behaviors.

- **Decrease Bullying Behaviors**

If your child gets bullied, help him or her to stand up to those who are bullying him or her and report the problem to the proper authorities.

- **Know the Warning Signs of Violence**

Be aware of the warning signs of violence and teach their children the signs as well.

- **Get Help When Needed**

Talk to your child's physician or nurse practitioner and get counseling for your child if he or she is showing problem behaviors.

*Adapted with permission from: Muscari, M. (2002). Not My Kid: 21 Steps to Raising a Nonviolent Child. Scranton, PA: University of Scranton Press. www.scrantonpress.com.*

# Internet Resources

## American Academy of Child and Adolescent Psychiatry
www.aacap.org
This Web site is an excellent source of information on the assessment and treatment of child and adolescent mental health disorders. Handouts for use with families (i.e., *Facts for Families*) are available on a multitude of problems, including conduct and oppositional defiant disorders.

## Early Warning Response, Timely Response: A Guide to Safe Schools
http://www.ed.gov/offices/OSERS/OSEP/Products/earlywrn.html
This is an excellent resource on how to create a safe environment in schools.

## KidsHealth
www.kidshealth.org
This is an outstanding Web site that contains health information for healthcare providers as well as excellent handouts for parents, teens, and children. Many of the topics relate to prevention of adverse health outcomes, including violence, and are developmentally sensitive to specific age groups. Physicians and other healthcare providers review all material before it is posted on this Web site.

## Sourcebook for Community Action
www.cdc.gov/ncipc/dvp/bestpractices.htm
This is a comprehensive guide on how to create safe communities.

## U.S. Surgeon General's Report on Youth Violence
www.surgeongeneral.gov/library/youthviolence
This report contains the best practices of youth violence prevention.

# References

American Psychiatric Association (2000). *Diagnostic and Statistical Manual of Mental Disorders, Fourth Edition* (DSM-IV). Washington, DC: APA.

Embry, D. (2001). Why more violent young offenders? *Corrections Today*, 63: 96-98.

Jellinek, M., Patel, B.P., & Froehle, M. (2002). *Bright Futures in Practice: Mental Health- Vol I. Practice Guide*. Arlington, VA: National Center for Education in Maternal and Child Health.

Jellinek, M., Patel, B.P., & Froehle, M. (2002). *Bright Futures in Practice: Mental Health- Vol II. Tool Kit*. Arlington, VA: National Center for Education in Maternal and Child Health.

Loeber, R. & Farrington, D. (1999). Etiology and delinquency predictions. Paper presented at Delinquents under 10: Targeting the Young Offender Conference at the University of Minnesota Law School Institute of Criminal Justice.

Melnyk, B.M., Brown, H., Jones, D.C., Kreipe, R., & Novak, J. (2003). Improving the mental/psychosocial health of U.S. children and adolescents. Outcomes and implementation strategies from the national KySS summit. *Journal of Pediatric Healthcare*, 17 (6: Supplement 1): S1- S24.

Wasserman, G., et al. (2003). Risk of protective factors of child delinquency. *Child Delinquency Bulletin Series, April*, 1-14. Office of Juvenile Justice and Delinquency Prevention.

# Reimbursement and Coding

Getting reimbursed for the time and effort that you spend caring for children with psychosocial and mental health issues requires a working knowledge of the diagnostic coding system and local practices of your third-party payers. The Current Procedural Terminology (CPT) coding book* is updated yearly and has thousands of diagnostic codes from which to choose. However, you may risk a rejected claim if your local insurers have restrictions on certain codes. In some areas, time-based codes for counseling can only be used by mental health providers, not by primary care providers. The list below is meant to save time from sorting through the entire CPT coding book, but you may want to ask your local insurance company if they recognize the code before you submit your bill.

## Routine Evaluation and Management Codes for Office Visits

The documentation guidelines established for each level need to be followed, including history of present illness, review of symptoms, past medical history, social history, physical exam, and medical complexity. These are the same codes used for "medical" office visits. For "established patients," the CPT codes are:

99211  level one, minimal severity
99212  level two, low severity
99213  level three, moderate severity
99214  level four,  high severity
99215  level five, very complex

## Time-Based Codes for Counseling

Documentation includes diagnosis and management as well as the time spent with the patient and/or family.

* Current Procedural Terminology (CPT) Coding Handbook by The American Medical Association.

For preventive medicine counseling and/or risk factor reduction:

| Individual | Group Visits |
|---|---|
| 99401 approximately 15 minutes | |
| 99402 approximately 30 minutes | 99411 approximately 30 minutes |
| 99403 approximately 45 minutes | |
| 99404 approximately 60 minutes | 99412 approximately 60 minutes |

The other part of appropriate billing involves attaching the proper diagnostic code (ICD-9 code).

These are some of the more common diagnoses that you will use when caring for the psychosocial needs of your pediatric patients:

| | |
|---|---|
| 300.0 | Anxiety state: unspecified |
| 300.02 | Generalized anxiety disorder |
| 300.9 | Suicide ideation |
| 300.4 | Dysthymia |
| 309.0 | Brief depressive reaction |
| 311 | Depressive disorder, chronic |
| 313.81 | Oppositional disorder |
| 309.24 | Adjustment disorder with anxious mood |
| 309.4 | Adjustment disorder with mixed emotions and conduct |
| 309.3 | Adjustment disorder with conduct disturbance |
| 309.0 | Adjustment disorder with depressed mood |
| 309.82 | Adjustment disorder with physical symptoms |
| 780.50 | Sleep disturbance, unspecified |
| 313.83 | Academic underachiever disorder |
| 314.01 | Attention deficit disorder with hyperactivity |
| 314.0 | Attention deficit disorder without hyperactivity |
| 278.01 | Obesity, morbid |
| 278.0 | Obesity, unspecified |
| 783.1 | Abnormal (excessive) weight gain |
| 783.21 | Weight loss |
| V65.5 | Feared condition not present |

## Information for Healthcare Providers about Brief Interventions

### What Are Brief Interventions

Brief interventions are counseling sessions delivered by primary care providers in the context of several standard office visits. These can be a successful treatment approach for many older school-age children and adolescents.

### Some Points of Brief Interventions

- Commonly used by clinicians to talk to patients about health issues or medication compliance
- Not unique to the alcohol field
- Designed for use in busy clinical settings
- Generally 5-10 minutes in duration
- Includes motivational interviewing and cognitive behavioral therapy (CBT) techniques
- More clinician-centered than client-centered therapy. Clinician shares concerns and tries to convince student to decrease alcohol use
- Uses an empathetic, nonconfrontational style
- Offers patient choices
- Emphasizes patient responsibility
- Conveys confidence in the patient's ability to change

*From: The National Institute on Alcohol Abuse and Alcoholism (NIAAA).*

# Introduction to Cognitive Behavior Skills Building

**Cognitive behavioral theory (CBT)** is rooted in cognitive theories that were developed by Ellis, Beck, and Seligman and in behavioral theories developed by Skinner and Lewinsohn. It suggests that irrational beliefs tend to cause individuals to overreact emotionally to certain precipitating events.

Beck proposed a negative cognitive triad of:

(a) a negative view of oneself, (b) one's environment, and (c) the future.

This pattern of thinking leads to hopelessness, anxiety, and depression.

Seligman's learned helplessness theory proposes that depression results from experiencing uncontrolled negative events with the belief that one cannot influence the outcomes with behavior.

A depressogenic cognitive thinking style includes internal attributions for negative events and external attributions for positive events.

Lewinsohn stressed that the lack of positive reinforcement from pleasurable activities/others leads to negative thought patterns.

Behavior theory suggests that individuals are depressed/anxious because of a lack of positive reinforcements and a lack of skills to elicit positive reinforcement from others or to terminate negative reactions from others.

**Antecedent Event:** Friends called me "chubbo"

**Belief:** I'm fat; I'll always be fat

**Emotional Outcome:** Depression

**Behavioral Outcome:** I give up; I won't try to eat healthy anymore

**Cognitive Behavior Skills Building**

CBT consists of cognitive restructuring (i.e., understanding the connection between thoughts and feelings as well as behaviors), problem solving, and behavioral change.

There is much evidence to support the effectiveness of CBT with depressed children and adolescents; CBT is labeled as probably effective for childhood anxiety disorders.

Homework is an essential component of CBT so that individuals can put into practice the skills that they are learning.

**Important: Individuals are taught that how they think is related to how they feel and how they behave (i.e., the thinking, feeling, behavior triangle).**

In CBT, individuals are taught to become aware of antecedent events as well as physical symptoms they are experiencing so that cognitive reappraisal and behaviors to reduce negative symptoms can be instituted early in the process.

Important skills in CBT are positive re-appraisal ("Okay, I'm not at my ideal weight, but with healthy eating and exercise, I can get there") and positive self-talk ("I can learn to eat healthy and exercise").

CBT should be conducted by mental health professionals who have in-depth education and skills to conduct this type of therapy. However, other professionals (e.g., primary care providers) can incorporate cognitive-behavior skills building in assisting children and teens to cope with stressors they are confronting in everyday life.

CBT should be practiced by mental health professionals with appropriate education and skills training; however, there are some key components of CBT that can be learned by health professionals to enhance children's and teens' abilities to cope with life stressors as well as to target symptoms of mild depression and anxiety.

The following segment (14.1) is an example of a segment from a brief CBT session by a healthcare provider (HP) with a depressed teen from the COPE/Healthy Lifestyles Program for Teens by Melnyk et al, 2004.

**The Clinical Case**

Anna is a 15-year-old girl who has been mildly depressed for the past few weeks, according to her mother. She does not want to go to her gymnastics class or hang out with her friends (new behaviors for her). Her appetite also has not been good lately. On interview, you find out that she received a D on a math test she took a couple of weeks ago, which seems to be a major cause of how she is feeling. It also did not help that a couple of her friends laughed at her score on the test.

During her interview, you discover that she believes that she is stupid, which is causing her to feel depressed and to not want to study anymore.

# Segment 14.1 - How People Change

| | |
|---|---|
| HP: Anna, I understand from your mom that you have been feeling down lately. | Anna: I sure have. |
| HP: On a scale of 0 to 10, with 0 meaning "not at all" to 10 meaning "a lot," how down or depressed have you been feeling over the past 2 weeks? | Anna: a 9. |
| HP: Anna- I'm going to continue to ask you some questions that will seem very personal, but all of the questions have to do with your health. What you tell me is confidential between the two of us, unless you tell me that you want to hurt yourself or that someone else has hurt you. Then, I need to tell another professional about it. I also want you to know that I ask all teens who are feeling down this questions. | Anna: Okay. |
| HP: Have you ever wished that you were dead or thought about hurting yourself? | Anna: Yes, one time -- last week. |
| HP: Did you think about how you would hurt yourself, that is, did you make a plan? | No, I really wouldn't ever try to kill myself because my parents would never forgive me. |
| HP: What do you think is causing you to feel so down lately? | Anna: I just feel I can't do anything right lately. A couple of weeks ago, I got a D on my math test when I studied for it. My close friends laughed at me, saying that I was getting dumber by the year. I don't even want to try anymore because I think "what's the use?" |
| HP: I can understand how you feel. I have felt the same way at times in my life, but you know what I found? Thinking like that only makes you feel down and depressed, and then you give up and don't try as hard. That only makes things worse. | Anna: I guess that's true, but I don't know what to do. Everything I do lately seems to go wrong. |
| HP: Anna, I could teach you a few tips on how you can start to feel better -- not so down. Do you want to hear about them? | Anna: Sure. |
| HP: There is something called the "thinking, feeling, behavior triangle." What that means is how you think affects how you feel and how you behave.<br>For instance, if something bad happens, like getting a D on your test, you believe that you are stupid, which makes you feel bad and not want to try anymore.<br>Can you think of another example? | Anna: Yeah. When my dad screams at me because I didn't clean my room, and I think "I flubbed up again," then I feel rotten about myself. |
| HP: That's right. Can you think of how you can turn that negative thought (i.e., "I flubbed up again") into a positive one? | Anna: Well, I guess I could think, "Okay, I put off cleaning my room, but that's okay; I'll get it done now." |
| HP: That's great, Anna. Now you are getting it. You have to start to monitor the way you are thinking when things happen and change the negative thought around as soon as it starts to happen into a positive thought, which will help you to feel a lot better. I'd like you to keep a log this week of all the things that happen that start making you have negative thoughts. I want you to write those down -- the event that happened that triggered you to have a negative thought -- and then, I want you write a positive thought that could replace the negative thought you had. Would you be willing to do that? | Anna: Sure, but do you really think this will help me? |
| HP: Yes, I do. It works for a lot of teens, and adults, too. When you come back, we'll work on more things and before you know it, you'll be feeling much better. | Anna: Okay, I'll try. |

For more examples of how cognitive-behavioral skills with teens can be built into clinical practice, please see the following downloadable resources.

*The Adolescent Coping with Stress Course (for teens at high risk for depression) and*
*The Adolescent Coping with Depression Course (for teens who are depressed), both available at*
http://www.kpchr.org/public/acwd/acwd.html

# Introduction to Motivational Interviewing

"Risky behaviors are a leading cause of preventable morbidity and mortality; yet behavioral counseling interventions to address them are underutilized in healthcare settings" (Whitlock, Orleans, Pender & Allan, 2002).

Motivational interviewing (MI) is a counseling intervention, based on Stages of Change Theory and Rogerian client-centered psychotherapy, which has been found to be effective in eliciting behavior change to promote health and reduce risk in adults. Evidence is accumulating to support similar effects of MI with adolescents (Sindelar, Abrantes, Hart, Lewander, & Spirito, 2004).

## What is Motivational Interviewing

MI is a "client-centered, directive method for enhancing intrinsic motivation to change by exploring and resolving ambivalence" (Miller & Rollnick, 2002). Originally, it was designed for multiple sessions of 30 minutes or longer, but MI has been adapted for brief (5-15 minute) encounters in a variety of settings.

## Essential Principles of Motivational Interviewing

- Express empathy
- Develop discrepancy
- Roll with resistance
- Support self-efficacy

## Spirit of Motivational Interviewing

- Readiness to change is a state (such as depression), not a trait (such as slow to adapt)
- Change comes from the client
- Resolving ambivalence is the client's task
- Helping client explore ambivalence
  — Avoid direct persuasion
  — Quiet, eliciting, respectful style
- Provider-client partnership

## How Do We Facilitate Change

Providers need to understand why people do change, do not change, and how they change.

## Why People Do Not Change

People don't change when the sum of the <u>forces discouraging</u> change is greater than the sum of the forces <u>encouraging</u> change (e.g., when what they like about smoking is greater than what they don't like about smoking, or their fear about quitting may be greater than the imagined of benefits of quitting).

## Why People Change

People change when the sum of the forces encouraging change is greater than the sum of the forces <u>discouraging</u> change (e.g., when the perceived negative consequences of drinking outweigh the benefits of drinking).

## How People Change

| Stages of Change | Intervention by Healthcare Provider |
|---|---|
| Pre-contemplation - not considering change | Increase awareness |
| Contemplation - considering change but ambivalent | Facilitate resolution of ambivalence |
| Preparation - willing to accept direction, anxious about change | Help client develop an action plan |
| Action - learning the new behavior | Solve problems related to new behavior |
| Maintenance - stable in the new behavior | Review successes, reinforce healthy behavior |
| Relapse - reappearance of old behavior - a process, not an event | Into action once again |

## Tools for Motivational Interviewing

* Agenda Setting - client determines priorities
  Example: "What would you like to talk about today...?"
* Getting Permission
  Example: "I'd like to spend a few minutes talking about...Is that okay with you?"
* Questions to get Started (open-ended)
  Example: "Tell me about..." "Help me understand..."
* Reflective Listening
  Example: "It sounds like you are feeling"; "It sounds like that is very important to you"
* Summarizing
  Examples: "What have I missed?"; "So it sounds like you have several reasons why you want to quit, but on the other hand there are things you like about smoking, that you aren't sure if you want to quit, or things you are worried about experiencing if you stop..."

- Eliciting Self-Motivational Statements: change talk
- Willing/Importance

    Example: "On a scale of 0 to 10 with 10 being very willing, how willing (interested, motivated) are you able to…(eat more fruits and vegetables, start using birth control...)?

    Example: "On a scale of 0 to 10 with 10 being very confident, assuming you decided to … (begin exercising, quit smoking), how <u>confident</u> are you that you could succeed?"

## Eliciting strengths and barriers

Example: "You said your confidence to change was 7. Why did you say 7 instead 0 or 1?"
Example: "You said your level of interest was 5. Why not 9 or 10?"

## Providing information without interpreting for the client

Example: "Chlamydia can increase a woman's risk of pelvic infections and infertility. What do you think about that?"

## Closing the deal

Example: "Where does that leave you?"  "Where do we go from here?"

## Markers of a Productive MI Encounter

- Client does most of the work
- Client accepts the possibility of change
- Client accepts the responsibility for change
- Upward slope of commitment language within or between sessions
- Dancing, not wrestling

## Clinical Case

Client is 16 years old, in clinic for a pregnancy test and STD check, history of multiple negative pregnancy tests and 1 case of Chlamydia in past year. The healthcare provider (HP) establishes rapport and updates history through a HEADSSS assessment, finding inconsistent condom use, no hormonal birth control, some alcohol and marijuana use, and an 8-month on-and-off consensual relationship with current boyfriend. (see Segment 14.2)

## Segment 14.2 - Clinical Case

| | |
|---|---|
| HP: Is there anything you want to talk about today? | Teen sets agenda |
| Teen: I want to find out if I'm pregnant. - I really don't want to be pregnant! | |
| HP: You really don't want be pregnant, so I think I have good news for you: your pregnancy test is negative.<br>I see we've done a few pregnancy tests for you this year. Can we talk about this a little? | Reflective listening<br>Getting permission |
| Teen: Okay, that's fine. | |
| HP: Tell me a little more about your condom use. | Open-ended question |
| Teen: We use them sometimes, when we have them, but I don't like to ask my boyfriend, and sometimes we're high, so we don't think about it. | |
| HP: So you really don't want to be pregnant, but sometimes you don't use condoms when you're high. What do you make of that? | Reflective listening<br>Developing discrepancy |
| Teen: Well I really haven't thought about that before. It sounds like I'm getting too relaxed and I'm not paying attention. | Teen is in pre-contemplation<br>Teen is interpreting information |
| HP: Let me ask you, on a scale of 0 to 10, where 0 is unimportant and 10 is very important, how important is condom use to you? | Eliciting change talk: willingness |
| Teen: I guess about a 7. | |
| HP: Why are you a 7 and not a 4? | Eliciting strengths |
| Teen: Well, I really don't want to be pregnant. | |
| HP: Okay. And what makes you a 7 and not a 9? | Eliciting barriers |
| Teen: Sometimes we don't have them, and I don't like asking him to put one on. | |
| HP: So sometimes you don't have condoms, and sometimes you don't like to ask about them. How confident are you in your ability to use condoms in the future, with 1 being not confident, and 10 being very confident? | Reflective listening<br>Eliciting change talk: self-efficacy |
| Teen: Around a 4. | |
| HP: Okay. What makes you a 4 and not a 1? | Eliciting strengths |
| Teen: Because we know how to use them and we do it sometimes. | |
| HP: Well, that's good. And what makes you a 4 and not a 7? | Supporting efficacy<br>Eliciting barriers |
| Teen: Well, sometimes I don't remember what I'm doing when I drink. | |
| HP: Well, I've heard you tell me that you don't want to be pregnant and that you and your boyfriend do use condoms, but that sometimes you don't have them and sometimes you don't remember when you drink. What do you think you might want to do now? | Reflective listening<br>Closing the deal |
| Teen: I guess I'd better not drink so much. I think I'm going to cut back on my drinking. | Teen is now in contemplation stage of change |

At this point, the HP would see if the teen is ready to commit to any definite actions, and help teen arrive at a plan.

# Tobacco Use among Children and Adolescents

According to the Clinical Practice Guidelines for Treating Tobacco Use and Dependence (Fiore et al., 2000), **parental tobacco use is the most significant predictor of youth smoking** (28. 5 % of high school students and 9.2% of middle school students currently smoke). Parents should be urged to stop smoking to prevent serious health implications for their children.

Tobacco dependence experts advocate screening all pediatric and adolescent patient *and* their parents for tobacco use. Clinicians should also advise children, adolescents, and parents to totally abstain from tobacco use.

Clinicians should assess adolescent tobacco use and offer tailored, developmentally appropriate interventions shown to be effective with adults, including developing a detailed quit plan (see http://www.surgeongeneral.gov/tobacco/tearsheet.pdf for a quit plan template), which includes strategies for coping with the challenges of cessation (especially withdrawal symptoms and social/emotional triggers to smoke) as well as the mobilization of intra and extra-treatment social support.

Additionally, adolescents may benefit from community and school-based intervention activities. Messages delivered through these venues should be reinforced by healthcare practitioners.

Clinicians in pediatric and adolescent practice settings should also educate parents about the health risks posed to their children from secondhand smoke.

Source: *Fiore M.C., Bailey, W.C., Cohen, S.J., et al. (2000).* Treating Tobacco Use and Dependence. Clinical Practice Guideline. *Rockville, MD: U. S. Department of Health and Human Services. Public Health Service.*

# Internet Resources

## Motivational Interviewing
www.motivationalinterview.org:
This Web site provides resources for those seeking information on motivational interviewing. It includes general information about the approach, as well as links, training resources, and information on reprints and recent research. In addition to providing information on motivational interviewing, the site serves as a resource for agencies or organizations who wish to find a skilled and knowledgeable trainer to assist them in implementing or supplementing current motivational services.

## National Institute on Alcohol Abuse and Alcoholism (NIAAA)
www.niaaa.nih.gov
This Web site has articles related to Brief Intervention interviewing, publications for consumers (easy-to-read material for the public covering a wide range of alcohol-related topics including "Publicaciones en Español"), publications for providers (treatment and prevention materials for healthcare providers and researchers), and a variety of other resources.

## National Institute of Drug Abuse (NIDA)
http://www.nida.nih.gov/TXManuals/CBT/CBT1.html
The NIDA has developed a series of "Therapy Manuals for Drug Addiction" series. The manuals present clear, helpful information to aid drug treatment practitioners in providing the best possible care. This link is specific to a manual on cognitive behavioral therapy (CBT) related to cocaine addition, but at the same time, provides an extensive overview of CBT and its use. The entire manual is available online, free of charge.

## The Centers for Disease Control and the Department of Health & Human Services offer the following resources aimed at helping youth who smoke to quit:

## Get Into Your Kid's Head. Here's how.
http://www.cdc.gov/tobacco/parenting/index.htm
DHHS, CDC
Getting more involved with your preteen or teen today will help you stay connected tomorrow. In addition, your involvement will help your child make better decisions. This brochure offers parents 10 specific methods for staying closer to their preteens or teens, such as scheduling weekly time and sharing meals. The brochure also suggests way to help teenagers quit smoking.

## The Tobacco-Free Sports Playbook: Pitching Healthy Lifestyles to Youth, Teams, and Communities
http://www.cdc.gov/tobacco/sports_initiatives.htm
CDC Manual: (2001) (6994)
This CDC guide is filled with information and examples of successful tobacco-free policies, media campaigns utilizing celebrity athletes, and education programs to help kids say "no" to tobacco and "yes" to better health. This easy-to-read guide was created to inspire kids to think about the many creative and effective ways they can incorporate sports and physical activity programs into tobacco-free activities.

## Individuals who wish to stop smoking may find the following resource helpful:
http://www.surgeongeneral.gov/tobacco/5dayplan.htm
You Can Quit Smoking. A 5-Day Plan To Get Ready. March 2001. U.S. Public Health Service.

# References on Motivational Interviewing

Motivational Interviewing: Resources for Clinicians, Researchers, and Trainers. Available at: www.motivationalinterview.org.

Emmons, K.M. & Rollnick, S. (2001). Motivational interviewing in health care settings: Opportunities and limitations. *American Journal of Preventive Medicine*, 20: 68-74.

Miller, W. R. & Rollnick, S. R. (2002). *Motivational Interviewing: Preparing People for Change (second edition)*. New York, NY: The Guilford Press.

Rustin, T.A. (2000). Facilitating Behavior Change. Keynote address at the 12th annual Texas Nurse Practitioners Conference in Austin, Texas.

Sindelar, H.A., Abrantes, A.M, Hart, C., Lewander, W., & Spirito, A. (2004). Motivational interviewing in pediatric practice. *Current Problems in Pediatric and Adolescent Health Care*, 34: 322-339.

Whitlock, E. P., Orleans, T., Pender, N., & Allan, J. (2002). Evaluating primary care behavioral counseling interventions: An evidence-based approach. *American Journal of Preventive Medicine*, 22: 267-284.

# References

Alloy, L.B., Peterson, C., Abramson, L.Y., & Seligman, M.E. Attributional style and the generality of learned helplessness. Journal of Personal and Social Psychology, 46 (3), 681-687.

Clarke GN, Hornbrook MC, Lynch F, Polen M, Gale J, Beardslee W, O'Connor E, Seeley J. A randomized trial of a group cognitive intervention for preventing depression in adolescent offspring of depressed parents. Archives of General Psychiatry 2001; 58(12).

Clarke GN, Rohde P, Lewinsohn PM, Hops H, Seeley JR. Cognitive-Behavioral Treatment of Adolescent Depression: Efficacy of Acute Group Treatment and Booster Sessions. Journal of the American Academy of Child and Adolescent Psychiatry 1999; 38(3):272-279.

DiClemente, C.C., Prochaska, J.O., Fairhurst, S.K., Velicer, W.F., Velasquez, M.M., Rossi, J.S. (1991). The process of smoking cessation: An analysis of precontemplation, contemplation and preparation stages of change. *Journal of Consulting and Clinical Psychology*, 59(2), 295-304.

Lewinsohn PM, Clarke GN, Hops H, Andrews J. Cognitive-behavioral group treatment of depression in adolescents. Behavior Therapy 1990; 21:385-401.

Melnyk, B.M., Small, L., Spath, L., & Morrison-Beedy. COPE/Healthy Lifestyles. An Intervention Program for Teens. Rochester, New York: COPE for HOPE, Inc.